SKELETAL MUSCLE IN HEALTH AND DISEASE

SKELETAL MUSCLE IN HEALTH AND DISEASE

A TEXTBOOK OF MUSCLE PHYSIOLOGY

D. A. Jones and J. M. Round

Manchester University Press

Manchester and New York

Distributed exclusively in the USA and Canada by St. Martin's Press

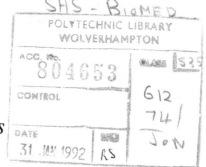

Copyright © D. A. Jones and J. M. Round 1990

Published by Manchester University Press
Oxford Road, Manchester M13 9PL

Distributed exclusively in the USA and Canada
by St. Martin's Press Inc.
175 Fifth Avenue, New York NY 10010, USA

British Library cataloguing in publication data
Jones, D. A. (David A.)
       Skeletal muscle in health and disease.
       1. Man. Muscles. Physiology
       I. Title   II. Round, Joan, M.
       612.74

Library of Congress cataloging in publication data
          Skeletal muscle in health and disease: a textbook of muscle
physiology / D. A. Jones and J. M. Round
           p. cm.
Includes bibliographical references.
ISBN 0-7190-3163-X. -- ISBN 0-7190-3164-8 (pbk.)
1. Muscles--Physiology. 2. Muscles--Diseases. I. Round, Joan M.
II. Title.
          [DNLM: 1. Muscles--Physiology.   WE 600 J76s]
QP321.J57 1990
612.7'4--dc20
DNLM/DLC
for Library of Congress   90-5631

ISBN   0-7190-3163-X *hardback*
ISBN   0-7190-3164-8 *paperback*

Printed in Great Britain
by Biddles Ltd, Guildford and King's Lynn

CONTENTS

PREFACE

For a number of years we have found it difficult to recommend any single textbook to students who are interested in muscle physiology, particularly in the area where exercise and clinical physiology overlap with the more conventional studies of isolated muscles and single fibres. This book is based on MSc, BSc and Sports Medicine courses which have been run in the Departments of Medicine and Physiology at University College during the last ten years and is intended to serve as a text for basic muscle physiology and to introduce topics that are of current research interest.

The first four chapters cover basic muscle structure, mechanics and the interactions of muscle and nerve. These topics are covered in many textbooks so we have concentrated on those aspects which we feel are often not clearly explained or illustrated. Some topics, notably the cardiovascular aspects of exercise, have not been included, primarily because they are well covered in most textbooks of human physiology. Chapters 5 to 10 concern training, growth, fatigue, damage and pain and include discussions of current and sometimes more controversial aspects of these subjects, based on our own experience and research. The final chapter is concerned with muscle diseases and we hope it will be an introduction to the subject for medical students and will also be of use to all who are interested in clinical physiology.

Being part textbook and part review it has been difficult to judge the extent to which references are required. At the end of each chapter there is a section entitled *References and further reading* which contains details of textbooks and review articles (often not specifically quoted in the text) to cover the broad generalisations, together with the specific references which have been cited in that chapter.

This text marks a new publishing venture in that the entire volume has been produced by the authors on a wordprocessor and we hope that it may encourage others to produce their own books tailored to the courses they teach. Teaching with an accompanying text must be a more efficient way of transmitting information than the usual inadequate system of note-taking by the students.

Finally we must thank our many present and former colleagues at the Hammersmith Hospital and University College who have helped to shape the overall view of skeletal muscle physiology presented here. Specifically we thank Caroline Sewery and Graham McPhail for providing the electron micrographs.

Chapter 1

SKELETAL MUSCLE STRUCTURE

Understanding the function of skeletal muscle requires a knowledge of its structure from the level of gross anatomy down to that of molecular organization.

Anatomy has always been the province of both medicine and art, the two coming together in the fifteenth century with the anatomical studies of Leonardo da Vinci, a tradition still maintained with art students working in the dissecting rooms of many of our Medical Schools. Study of the fine structure of muscle also has a long and interesting history with the banded appearance of skeletal muscles first being described by Van Leeuwenhock in the 1670s. During the nineteenth century knowledge of fine structure advanced rapidly with the improvements in optics and staining techniques which took place during what has been described as the "golden age" of microscopy. In the first half of the twentieth century, however, studies of structure were overshadowed by advances in biochemistry and physiology, and many relevant observations made by nineteenth century microscopists such as Bowman and Dobie in England and Krause in Germany were largely forgotten. It was not until the 1950s, with the renewed interest in light microscopy and the use of the electron microscope to examine sarcomere structure and the organisation of the contractile filaments, that the study of structure again became of primary importance to our understanding of muscle function.

The structure of muscle needs to be understood from the molecular organisation of the contractile proteins to the macroscopic arrangement of fibres, connective tissue and tendons. The description that follows begins with the contractile proteins, explains how these are arranged into sarcomeres and myofibrils within muscle fibres and then how the fibres combine with connective tissue to form the whole muscle.

1.1 The contractile proteins

Deliberate movement is one of the features that separates animal from plant life and clearly the contractile proteins play an important role in this process. Nevertheless, contractile proteins, especially actin, are found in all types of cell, being responsible for protoplasmic streaming and the movement of intracellular organelles. Actin is a protein of great antiquity and is highly conserved in the sense that actins from animal and plant cells are functionally and immunologically very similar. Skeletal and cardiac muscle are unusual, not so much for possessing actin and myosin, but for their particularly high content (about 80% of the total protein) and for having these two proteins arranged in a highly ordered array within the cell permitting the controlled generation of force and movement.

1.1.1 *Actin*

Actin is a globular protein (g actin) with a molecular weight of 42,000 which polymerizes into what appear to be double helical strands (f actin) (Fig. 1.1; Cohen & Vibert, 1987, for a general review). The apparent double-stranded structure may be artifactual as recent evidence suggests that the actin monomer is bilobed and, when polymerised, gives the impression of a double helical structure (Korne *et al*, 1987). The polymerization of actin involves splitting ATP and the binding of ADP. About 90% of the ADP in muscle is bound to actin. The actin filaments (also known as *thin filaments*) are variable in length with mammalian filaments being somewhat longer than those of amphibian muscle. The thin filament length also varies between muscles of the same animal and even within a sarcomere so that the edge of the I band (see Fig. 1.4) is somewhat irregular.

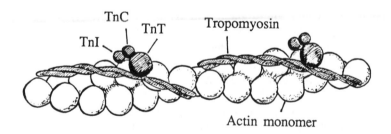

Fig. 1.1 Part of an actin filament together with tropomyosin and the troponin subunits.

Tropomyosin and the three troponin subunits TnC, TnT and TnI, form the other constituents of the thin filaments (Fig. 1.1). The tropomyosin extends over seven actin subunits and blocks the myosin binding sites until caused to move by calcium binding to troponin C. The periodicity of the troponin subunits along the thin filament has been demonstrated by staining with antibodies to troponin T showing between 24 and 30 repeats depending on the length of the thin filaments.

The actin filaments join at one end to form the Z line structure (Fig. 1.2). At the Z line the actin filaments are in a square array with each thin filament in one half sarcomere being linked to four other filaments in the next half sarcomere. The protein α-actinin forms the connections between the actin filaments (Franzini-Armstrong, 1973).

In fast muscles the linkage is quite simple giving a thin Z line, while in slow fibres there may be several connections between the two sets of thin filaments giving a thicker Z line (see Fig. 1.11).

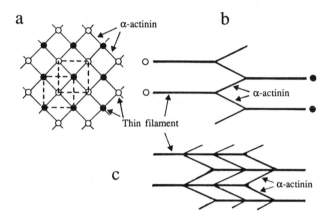

Fig. 1.2 Actin filaments joining to form the Z line. **a**, view of the Z line along the axis of the thin filaments showing the square array. Solid symbols indicate thin filaments coming out of the page (or Z line), open symbols thin filaments going into the page. **b**, view from the side; note that only the α-actinin connections in the plane of the page are shown, for every thin filament there will be another two connections in a plane at right angles to the page. **b** represents a simple Z line structure found in fast muscle. **c**, more complex Z line found in slow skeletal and cardiac muscle.

1.1.2 *Myosin*

Myosin molecules consist of two identical chains, each with a molecular weight of approximately 200,000, together with four light chains each of around 20,000 molecular weight (Knight & Trinick, 1987, for a general review). In mollusc muscle the myosin light chains have a clear regulatory role, binding calcium and controlling the activity of myosin. Mammalian light chains can substitute for mollusc light chains, demonstrating that they have functional potential but, to date, no unequivocal role for these proteins has been found in mammalian muscle. The composition of the light chains differs between fast and slow muscles.

The myosin molecule can be split enzymatically into a number of fragments (Fig. 1.3a & 1.3b). The globular head, or S1 fragment,

contains the enzymic activity and is the portion that can combine with
actin. The S2 portion is a flexible region of the molecule, while the
tail (light meromyosin, LMM) combines with other tails, binding the
myosin molecules together to form the *thick filaments* (Fig. 1.3c). Thick
filaments consist of approximately 300 molecules arranged so that the
myosin heads are pointing in one direction at one end of the filament
and in the opposite direction at the other end. Consequently there is a
region in the centre of each filament where there are only tails and no
projecting heads. This region constitutes about 10% of the total length.
Unlike the thin filaments, which can vary, the thick filaments are very
uniform in length throughout the animal kingdom (Offer, 1987).

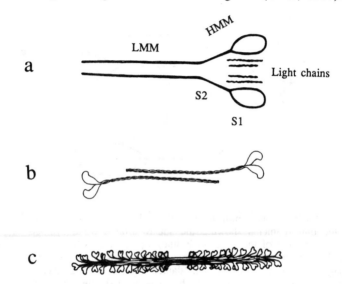

Fig. 1.3 Myosin structure and assembly into thick filaments. **a**, schematic arrangement
of myosin subunits. **b** & **c**, the basic double headed myosin units aggregating to form
a thick filament.

The thick myosin filaments are arranged so that the thin actin
filaments, attached to the Z lines, can slide between (Fig. 1.4). The
unit from Z line to Z line is known as a sarcomere and, in mammalian
muscle held at a resting length in the body, is between 2 and 2.5µm
long. Each thick filament is surrounded by six thin filaments (Fig. 1.4).
At the Z lines the thin filaments are held in a square array whereas in
the overlap region they are forced into a hexagonal array by the
arrangement of the thick filaments. The thin filaments must, therefore,
be somewhat flexible and in the I band region where there is no overlap,
they have a no regular array (Squire *et al*, 1987, for a general review of
the myofibril structure).

The nomenclature of the various bands in a sarcomere is shown in Fig. 1.4. The A and I bands are so called because of their birefringent properties under the light microscope, the I band being isotropic and the A band anisotropic. At a more mundane level the bands can be remembered as being light (I) and dark (A) when seen in longitudinal sections with the electron microscope. The area in the A band where there is no overlap with thin filaments is known as the H zone in the centre of which is the region of the thick filaments bare of projecting myosin heads. Proteins running across this region give rise to the M line (see Section 1.2).

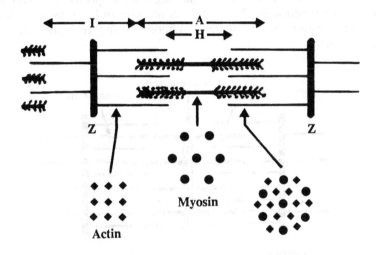

Fig. 1.4 The arrangement of thick and thin filaments to form a sarcomere. Below; cross-sections of the sarcomere.

Identification of the two contractile proteins and understanding how they are arranged to give the banded appearance of skeletal muscle has been central to an understanding of the mechanism of force generation. This knowledge has been derived, first, from observations with the light microscope showing that the A band is of a constant width, while it is the I band that changes as the muscle lengthens and contracts. Secondly, careful observations at the electron microscope level of the way in which myosin monomers in solution aggregate to form the characteristic bidirectional filaments, indicated the structure and possible function of the thick filaments (Fig. 1.3c). Thirdly, the location of the different proteins was confirmed by elegant experiments in which myosin was extracted from dissociated myofibrils with KCl solution containing ATP or pyrophosphate, showing that, after extraction, the Z line and I bands remained but the A band had been removed.

1.2 Structural proteins

There are a variety of proteins whose function is probably to maintain the architecture of the sarcomere (Fig. 1.5). Proteins in the M line keep the myosin filaments in the correct spatial arrangement for the actin filaments to slide between them. The thick filaments have a banded appearance which is enhanced by staining with a specific antibody to C protein. The function of this protein is not known but may be involved in the aggregation of the myosin monomers and regulation of thick filament length.

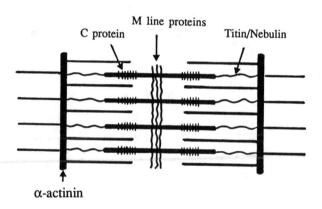

Fig. 1.5 Structural proteins in the sarcomere.

Titin is an extremely long protein molecule (about 1μm) that links the myosin filaments to the Z line. The value of such a connection is to keep the A band located in the centre of the sarcomere at times when the sarcomere is stretched to lengths where there is little or no overlap of the thick and thin filaments. Nebulin is another very large protein found associated with actin near the Z line, but whose function is not known.

α-actinin forms part of the Z line structure binding the actin filaments together and *desmin* links the Z lines of adjacent myofibrils (see below) and serves to keep the Z lines in register. *Spectrin* and *dystrophin* are proteins that probably have a structural role in the surface membrane of the muscle fibre.

1.3 The myofibril

Bundles of 100-400 thick filaments form *myofibrils* which are separated one from another by sarcoplasmic reticulum, T tubules (see below) and sometimes mitochondria. Myofibrils vary in size but average around 1μm in diameter and make up about 80% of the volume of a muscle fibre. The numbers of myofibrils vary with the size of the muscle fibre and can be as few as 50 in a developing foetal muscle fibre. There are about 2000 myofibrils in an adult muscle fibre.

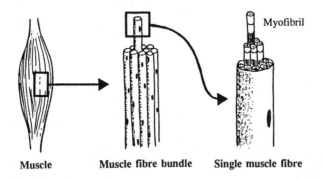

Myofibril

Muscle   **Muscle fibre bundle**   **Single muscle fibre**

Fig. 1.6 Diagramatic representation of the relationship between the muscle, muscle fibres and myofibrils. In reality the myofibrils are very much smaller, in relation to the muscle fibre, than shown here.

1.4 Sarcoplasmic reticulum

Each myofibril is enveloped in a complex membranous bag, the interior of which is quite separate from the cytoplasm of the fibre (Fig. 1.7).

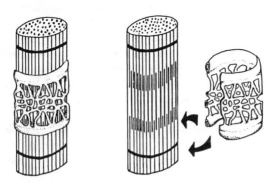

Fig. 1.7 The sarcoplasmic reticulum envelops a myofibril.

The membrane system is known as the sarcoplasmic reticulum and acts as a store for the uptake and release of calcium (Peachey, 1965). The portions near the T tubules (see Section 1.6) are known as the terminal cisternae. In fast muscle fibres the sarcoplasmic reticulum may surround each myofibril, but in slower fibres the membrane system is less well developed (Eisenberg, 1983).

1.5 T-tubular system

The plasma membrane of the muscle fibre invaginates to form a complex tubular system which forms a branching network running across the whole fibre and contacting every myofibril (Fig. 1.8).

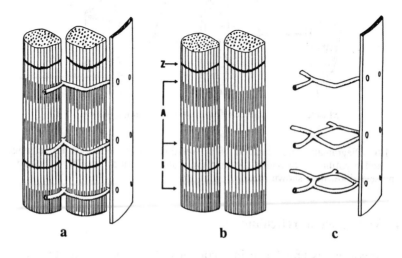

Fig. 1.8 The T tubules in relation to the sarcomere. T tubules invaginate from the surface membrane of the muscle fibre (**c**) and contact the myofibrils at the junction of the A and I band (**a** & **b**).

The invaginations of the surface membrane occur twice in every sarcomere approximately at the level of the junction of the A and I bands. In amphibian muscle, in contrast to mammalian muscle, there is only one T tubule per sarcomere and this runs at the level of the Z line.

Where the T tubules meet the sarcoplasmic reticulum the two membranes are closely applied (Fig. 1.9) and electron dense "feet" have been described linking the two sets of membranes (see Chapter 3, Section 3.4).

In electron micrograph sections the T tubules are often seen cut in cross section with a portion of the sarcoplasmic reticulum on either side

(Figs. 1.9 & 10), this is known as a "triad". When associated with sarcoplasmic reticulum in a triad the T tubule is flattened, otherwise it tends to be circular in cross section.

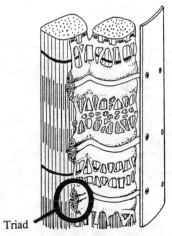

Triad

Fig. 1.9   T tubules, sarcoplasmic reticulum and the myofibrils.   Insert shows the structure of a triad.

If a muscle is incubated in a solution containing an electron dense substance such as ferritin, particles are found in the lumen of the T tubules (Page, 1964). This observation demonstrates that the T tubules are continuous with the extracellular fluid. No diffusion of ferritin into the sarcoplasmic reticulum is seen, showing that the lumen of the sarcoplasmic reticulum is not continuous with that of the T tubular system, although their membranes are closely associated.

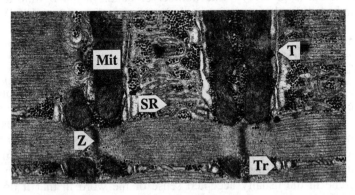

Fig. 1.10   EM of mouse fast muscle showing the appearance of T tubules and sarcoplasmic reticulum surrounding the myofibril. The section has grazed the surface of the upper myofibril showing the membrane structures. **T**, T tubule; **Tr**, Triad; **Z**, Z line; **Mit**, mitochondria; **SR**, sarcoplasmic reticulum.

1.6 The EM appearance of different fibre types

There is considerable interest in the possibility of identifying different fibre types by their EM appearances.

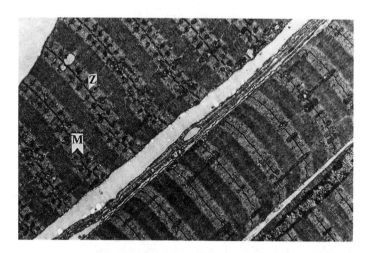

Fig. 1.11 EM of two adjacent mouse muscle fibres; top, slow type 1 fibre with thick Z lines (**Z**) and numerous mitochondria (**M**); below fast type 2 fibre with thinner Z line and few mitochondria.

A number of features have been claimed to distinguish fast from slow fibres, including the width of the Z line and density of mitochondria (Fig. 1.11). The number of bands in the M line are also reported to differ between fast and slow fibres (Eisenberg, 1983).

1.7 Muscle organisation

Each muscle fibre is bounded by its sarcolemma. The innermost portion of the sarcolemma is the plasma membrane which is the true boundary of the cell. At resting lengths the plasma membrane is folded with small indentations or *caveolae*. These smooth out as the muscle is stretched and are probably important in allowing considerable change in muscle fibre length without causing damage to the surface membrane. Outside the plasma membrane is the basement membrane which not a membrane in the usually accepted sense of the word in that it does not have a lipid bilayer structure but is composed of a loose glycoprotein and collagen network. It is freely permeable and may surround more than one fibre. Following muscle fibre damage the basement membrane forms a framework within which regeneration occurs.

Adult muscle fibres vary considerably in size and length between various muscles in the body and between individuals of different sex, build and age. In a normal adult the mean cross-sectional fibre areas are between $2500\mu m^2$ (small woman) and $7500\mu m^2$ (large man), representing a variation in diameter of about 50-100μm. Fibres from a muscle such as the quadriceps are on average larger, in any individual, than fibres from smaller muscles such as the masseter or muscles of the hand. Fibre length varies greatly, from a few millimetres in the ciliary muscles of the eye to 10cm or more in the sartorius, a long, strap-like muscle in the inner thigh.

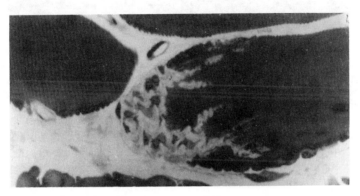

Fig. 1.12 Myotendinous junction. Low power EM.

At the ends of a muscle fibre the outer membranes become irregular and indented to form a close link with the connective tissue (Fig. 1.12). The connective tissue elements all come together to form the tendons which join the muscle to the bony skeleton.

Between the muscle fibres are fibroblasts which secrete collagen fibres to form a thin connective tissue matrix, the endomysium. Groups of 10 to 100 muscle fibres are surrounded by a thicker layer of connective tissue, the perimysium, to form fascicles (Fig. 1.13).

Small blood vessels and motor axons traverse the perimysial spaces to make connections with the muscle fibres. Muscle spindles are also found enclosed in connective tissue envelopes in the perimysium. Each muscle is covered by a thick outer connective tissue layer, the epimysium.

Fibroblasts, and their major product collagen, play an important role maintaining both the structure of a muscle and an environment within which the contractile muscle fibre can function. However, just as glial cells have, in the past, been overlooked in neurophysiology so fibroblasts are the Cinderella cells of muscle physiology, most attention going to the more flamboyant, contractile, muscle fibres.

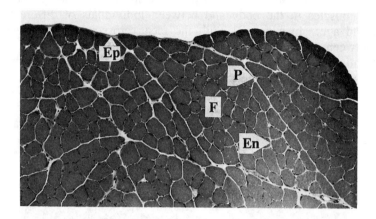

Fig. 1.13   Transverse section through a portion of mouse skeletal muscle.   Light microscope; section stained with haematoxylin and eosin. **F**, fascicle; **En**, endomysium; **P**, perimysium; **Ep**, epimysium.

In the average quadriceps muscle there are about one million fibres in a section taken at the mid-thigh level (Fig. 1.14), however, the muscle has a complex structure so that a single cross section will not include all the fibres, and the whole muscle may consist of several million fibres.

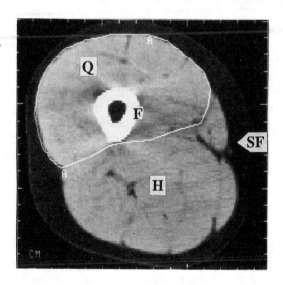

Fig. 1.14   Cross-section through the human mid-thigh.   Section obtained by computerised tomography and shows the quadriceps (**Q**) and hamstring (**H**) muscles together with the femur (**F**) and subcutaneous fat (**SF**).

1.8 **Other microscopic structures**

1.8.1 *Mitochondria*

Mitochondria are a prominent feature of muscle fibres when viewed with the electron microscope (Fig. 1.15). They are seen just below the plasma membrane (subsarcolemmal) and between the myofibrils where they tend to be situated on either side of the Z lines between the T tubules of adjacent sarcomeres (see also Fig. 1.10). This proximity to the extracelluar fluid within the T tubules may be useful in keeping diffusion distances for oxygen to a minimum. The number of mitochondria within a fibre can vary considerably, slow oxidative fibres containing more than fast fibres (Eisenberg, 1983).

1.8.2 *Glycogen granules*

Glycogen granules are seen as small black dots in EM photographs (Fig. 1.15); they appear to be packed between myofibrils wherever the space is not occupied by sarcoplasmic reticulum or mitochondria. The number of granules varies not only between fast and slow fibres but also with nutritional status and whether or not the muscle has been depleted of glycogen by sustained activity.

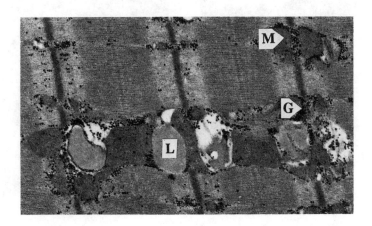

Fig. 1.15 Mitochondria, glycogen and lipid in a muscle fibre. **M**, mitochondria; **G**, glycogen granules; **L**, lipid droplet.

1.8.3 *Lipid droplets*

Lipid droplets (Fig. 1.15) are occasionally seen in endomysial areas between normal fibres and very small lipid droplets are also seen within muscle fibres. Type 1 fibres contain more fine droplets of fat than do type 2 fibres. Lipid droplets often dissolve during staining procedures leaving small unstained holes. Deposition of lipid in both intracellular and extracelluar areas can become extensive in some diseases such as Duchenne muscular dystrophy (Chapter 11, Section 11.3).

1.8.4 *Muscle fibre nuclei*

Muscle fibres are multinucleate cells. The nuclei lie at the periphery of the fibres just below the plasma membrane (Fig. 1.16a). In a cross-section of a muscle between 4-10μm thick viewed with a light microscope, two or three nuclei per fibre can normally be seen, thus it can be estimated that there are about 200 to 300 nuclei per mm of muscle fibre length.

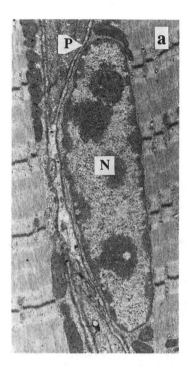 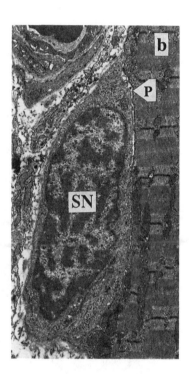

Fig. 1.16 Muscle fibre nucleus and satellite cell. **a**, muscle fibre nucleus (**N**) just below the plasma membrane (**P**). **b**, satellite cell lying outside the muscle plasma membrane with a layer of cytoplasm around the nucleus; **SN**, satellite cell nucleus.

1.8.5 *Satellite cells*

Satellite cells, derived from embryonic myoblasts lie between the plasma membrane and the basement membrane of muscle fibres. Each satellite cell consists of a large nucleus with a thin layer of cytoplasm and they cannot be distinguished from the nuclei of the muscle fibres when viewed with a light microscope. Using an electron microscope, satellite cells can be identified by their position outside the plasma membrane but beneath the basement membrane of the muscle fibre (Fig. 1.16b).

If the muscle fibre is damaged, satellite cells are activated and initiate regeneration (Chapter 9, Section 9.4).

1.8.6 *Muscle spindles*

Muscle spindles are complex receptor organelles containing several small specialised muscle fibres which have both an afferent and efferent nerve supply. These fibres are known as *intrafusal* fibres in contrast to the *extrafusal* fibres in the bulk of the muscle. The whole structure is enclosed in a connective tissue capsule filled with lymph. There are two types of intrafusal muscle fibre in a spindle, larger *nuclear bag* fibres and small *nuclear chain* fibres.

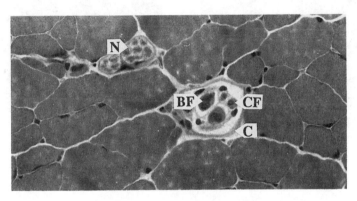

Fig. 1.17 Muscle spindle. **C**, capsule; **BF**, bag fibre; **CF**, chain fibre; **N**, small nerve bundle.

Transverse sections in the equatorial region of a spindle (Fig. 1.17) show nuclear bag fibres with several grouped nuclei and chain fibres with apparently only a single nucleus, the other nuclei being above and below the plane of the section in a chain formation. Muscle spindles provide sensory information about the absolute length and the rate of length change of a muscle (Chapter 4, Section 4.6.2).

1.8.7 *Neuromuscular junction*

Neuromuscular junctions are not often seen in EM preparations from biopsy material as there is only one junction per fibre and the chances of sectioning this region are small. The appearance is of very irregular infoldings of the muscle plasma membrane and there is often an accumulation of glycogen and mitochondria just beneath the junction (Fig. 1.18 a,b).

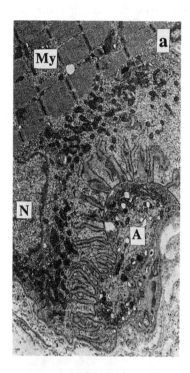 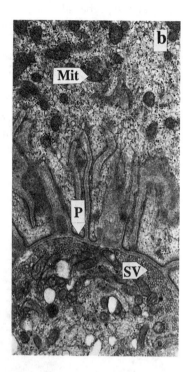

Fig. 1.18 Neuromuscular junction. **a**, low power EM; **A**, nerve axon; **P**, muscle fibre plasma membrane; **N**, nucleus; **My**, myofibrils. **b**, higher power EM; **SV**, synaptic vesicles; **Mit**, muscle mitochondria.

1.8.8 *Lipofuchsin deposits*

Lipofuchsin deposits are sometimes seen in EM photographs of normal muscle and are thought to be the products of degraded membrane lipids. Lipofuchsin is often described as an ageing pigment as deposits are more commonly seen in muscle from the elderly.

1.9 References and further reading

Cohen, C. & Vibert, P.J. (1987). Actin filament: images and models. In: *Fibrous Protein Structure*, ed. J.M. Squire & P.J. Vibert. London, Academic Press, pp. 284-306.

Craig, R. & Offer, G. (1976). The location of C-protein in rabbit skeletal muscle. *Proceedings of the Royal Society London* B **192**, 451-61.

Eisenberg, B.R. (1983). Quantitative ultrastructure of mammalian skeletal muscle. In: *Handbook of Physiology, Section 10, Skeletal muscle.* ed. L.D. Peachey, R.H. Adrian & S.R. Geiger, Bethesda, American Physiological Society, pp. 73-112.

Franzini-Armstrong, C. (1973). The structure of a simple Z line. *Journal of Cell Biology* **58**, 630-42.

Hanson, J. & Huxley, H.E. (1955). The structural basis of contraction in striated muscle. *Symposia of the Society for Experimental Biology* **IX**, pp. 228-64.

Huxley, A.F. (1976). Looking back on muscle. In: *The Pursuit of Nature.* Cambridge, Cambridge University Press, pp. 23-64.

Knight, P. & Trinick, J. (1987). The myosin molecule. In: *Fibrous Protein Structure*, ed. J.M. Squire & P.J. Vibert. London, Academic Press, pp. 247-81.

Korne, D., Carlier, M.F. & Ptaloni, D. (1987). Actin polymerisation and ATP hydrolysis. *Science*, **238**, 638-44.

Needham, D. (1971). *Machina Carnis.* Cambridge, Cambridge University Press.

Offer, G. (1987). Myosin filaments. In: *Fibrous Protein Structure*, ed. J.M. Squire & P.J. Vibert. London, Academic Press, pp. 307-56.

Ohtsuki, I. (1975). Distribution of troponin components in the thin filament studied by immunoelectron microscopy. *Journal of Biochemistry* **77**, 633-39.

Page, S.G. (1964). The organisation of the sarcoplasmic reticulum in frog muscle. *Journal of Physiology* **175**, 10P-11P.

Page, S.G. & Huxley, H.E. (1963). Filament lengths in striated muscle. Journal of Cell Biology **19**, 369-90.

Peachey, L.D. (1965). The sarcoplasmic reticulum and transverse tubules of the frog's sartorius. *Journal of Cell Biology* **25**, Suppl. 3, 209-31.

Squire, J.M, Luther, P.K. & Trinick, J. (1987). Muscle myofibril architecture. In: *Fibrous Protein Structure*, ed. J.M. Squire & P.J. Vibert. London, Academic Press, pp. 423-50.

Chapter 2

THE MECHANISM OF FORCE GENERATION

In discussing muscle structure and the generation of force the impression is frequently given that current ideas about the action of cross bridges arose naturally from observations of the structure and composition of the thick filaments and their position in relation to the actin filaments. However, the interpretation of microscopic, EM and X-ray evidence is inevitably influenced by conceptual models based on the mechanical properties of muscle, and current ideas have evolved as a result of the interaction between workers investigating the mechanical properties of contracting muscle and those exploiting the advantages of visualizing the actin and myosin filaments. Since the 1950s the commanding figures in this dialogue have been A.F. Huxley and H.E. Huxley.

In this chapter the mechanical properties of contracting muscle are presented together with a discussion of the evidence that these properties provide about the nature of the mechanism for generation of force in skeletal muscle.

2.1 Methods for measuring contractile properties

Amphibian and mammalian muscles can be studied either *in situ* with one tendon attached to a bone and the other to a strain gauge, or whole muscles can be dissected out and incubated in a temperature-controlled bath for *in vitro* studies. Amphibian muscles are usually maintained at 0°C and mammalian muscles at around 25°C; these temperatures are generally chosen for convenience and to maintain tissue viability rather than for any physiological reasons.

Much of the crucial work on muscle mechanics has involved the use of single-fibre preparations generally obtained from amphibian muscles. Dissection of single frog fibres is difficult and it is very difficult to obtain viable single mammalian fibres as they are more securely held together with connective tissue. Small bundles of fibres are conveniently prepared from rabbit psoas muscle or from the flight muscles of some larger insects. The surface membrane can be removed by storing the preparations in a solution of glycerol.

Length-tension relationships can be demonstrated in isolated muscle preparations using a simple apparatus with which to stimulate the muscle and record isometric force. To take these observations further and relate force to the structure of the sarcomere, a method of measuring sarcomere length is required. If laser light is directed at a thin muscle preparation the regular sarcomere pattern acts as a diffraction grating which can be used to determine sarcomere spacing (Fig 2.1). Problems arise because sarcomeres may not be uniform along the length of the muscle fibre. This difficulty can be partly overcome by using short preparations and a feedback system which monitors the length of a fibre segment and adjusts the preparation to keep this length constant.

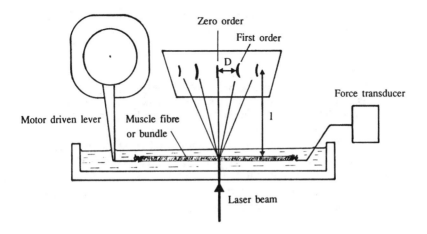

Fig. 2.1 Apparatus to measure force/velocity characteristics of small fibre bundles and single fibres. Also shown is the measurement of sarcomere spacing using diffraction of laser light. Sarcomere spacing = $\lambda/\sin\theta$ where λ is the wavelength of the light and θ the angle subtended by the first order diffraction line, $\tan\theta = D/l$.

The force-velocity properties of muscle were first characterised in the 1920s and 1930s using lever systems to load the contracting muscle, but these methods have now been replaced largely by devices in which controlled movement is produced by a stepping motor, the moving arm of a pen recorder motor or the coil of a loudspeaker (Fig. 2.1). With appropriate feedback control these systems can be used either for constant velocity (*isokinetic*) or constant force (*isotonic*) contractions. A record of isokinetic shortening is shown in Fig. 2.2.

The maximum velocity of shortening (Vmax) can be estimated by extrapolating the velocities measured for smaller and smaller loads but is often uncertain because the curve approaches the velocity axis at a narrow angle. An alternative way of estimating Vmax is the so called "slack" test.

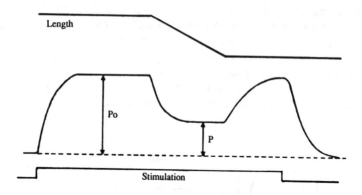

Fig. 2.2 Record of isokinetic shortening. The muscle is held at a fixed length whilst isometric tension develops (Po) and is then released at a constant velocity. Measurements of force (P) are made once a steady state has been reached.

A contracting muscle is rapidly shortened by a known distance (at a velocity greater than Vmax) so that the fibres become slack and will then shorten with no external load. The time for the fibre to take up the slack and begin pulling on the force transducer gives a measure of the velocity of unloaded shortening (Fig. 2.3).

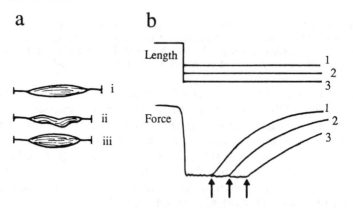

Fig. 2.3   Slack test to establish maximum velocity of shortening. a, i, muscle contracting isometrically; ii, muscle rapidly released; iii, muscle shortens, takes up slack and redevelops tension. b, muscle released for three different lengths. The time to begin redeveloping tension (arrow) on the coresponding force record is used to calculate the velocity of unloaded shortening.

2.2 Length-tension relationship of skeletal muscle

There are two components of the total force that can be measured: the *passive tension* which is due to stretching the connective tissue elements of the muscle and, possibly, the structural protein titin. The *active tension* is superimposed on the passive tension when the muscle is stimulated (Fig 2.4). In the discussion that follows we are concerned only with the active tension, the passive component being subtracted from the total force.

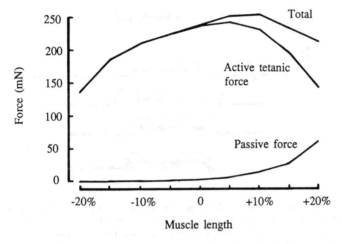

Fig. 2.4 The two components of force, passive and active tension. Total force is the sum of the two components. Mouse soleus muscle, 26°C, stimulated at 100Hz.

The main feature of the length-tension relationship is that force declines on either side of an optimum length and, by extrapolating the line at longer lengths, a value can be predicted at which no tension would be generated. It is not possible to stretch most whole muscles far enough, but some frog and toad muscles can be extended this far.

If force is generated by the interaction of actin and myosin this should vary according to the degree of overlap of these two sets of filaments. Knowing the lengths of the filaments it is possible to predict the length-tension relationship and the sarcomere length at which no force would be developed. Taking care to keep the sarcomere lengths constant by length clamping segments of the muscle fibre, Gordon *et al* (1966) found a close fit between the actual and predicted force (Fig. 2.5). These results constitute one of the foundations of the cross-bridge theory, demonstrating that force is generated by the interaction of the overlapping portions of actin and myosin filaments and this is known as the sliding filament theory of contraction.

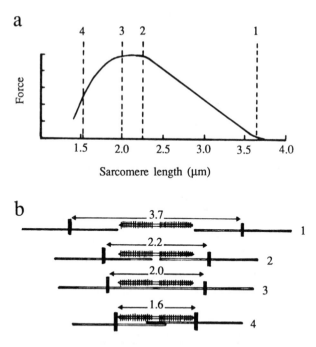

Fig. 2.5   Isometric force at different sarcomere lengths.   **a** force generated; **b**, arrangement of filaments at different lengths.   At lengths less than 2.0μm thin filaments begin to overlap and at still shorter lengths the thick filaments come into contact with the Z lines.   Values are for frog muscle (redrawn from Gordon *et al*, 1969); mammalian thin filaments are slightly longer so the corresponding sarcomere lengths are 1 - 4.0μm, 2 - 2.5μm, 3 - 2.4μm and 4 - 1.6μm.

Unless great care is taken to keep sarcomere lengths constant a significant discrepancy is observed between the actual and predicted values for the right-hand descending limb of the length tension curve. Force is still developed at sarcomere lengths where no filament overlap would be expected (Fig. 2.6a).

The reason for the difference between observed and predicted results lies in the phenomenon generally known as "creep". Close examination of the single fibre preparations used in this type of work shows that the sarcomere spacing is not uniform along the length of a fibre, the sarcomeres at the ends of the fibre being shorter than those in the middle (Fig. 2.6b). If the muscle is set to a long length so that, in the majority of sarcomeres, the filaments are just overlapping then, during contraction, the sarcomeres at the ends of the fibre will be shorter and generate more force. In doing so the end sarcomeres will shorten further at the expense of the sarcomeres in the centre and the force will gradually "creep" up. The right-hand limb of the length tension relationship will appear to have an intercept further along the length axis than would be expected.

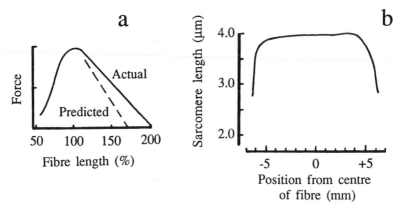

Fig. 2.6 Variations in sarcomere length along a muscle fibre and the phenomenon of creep. **a**, difference between actual force and that predicted from filament lengths showing more force than expected at longer lengths (Ramsey & Street, 1940). **b**, sarcomere lengths along the length of a fibre. Note the shorter sarcomeres at the ends of the fibre (Gordon *et al*, 1966).

It is not known why sarcomeres at the ends of the fibre should be more resistant to extension than those at the centre. This behaviour also raises an interesting question as to how force is transmitted through the central sarcomeres when there is apparently little or no overlap of actin and myosin filaments (see Section 2.4.4).

2.3 The nature of the interaction between thick and thin filaments

Over the years various ideas have been put forward about the nature of the actin and myosin interaction. As well as the cross-bridge theory there have also been models in which force is generated by actin and myosin forming helical structures (e.g. Astbury, 1950). Observations such as those first made by Gasser & Hill (1924) showed that if an active muscle is allowed to shorten rapidly by as little as 1% of its total length, the force generated momentarily drops to near zero before redeveloping. If the actin and myosin had formed into some kind of long spring when the muscle was activated the force would be expected to decrease roughly in proportion to the change in its overall length, that is, it would obey Hooke's law. A 1% decrease in length for a long spring would be expected to drop the force by 1%, not the value close to 100% that is observed. This important observation suggests that force is generated by components which are very short, so that a change of 1% of the sarcomere length is sufficient to take all the stretch out of them (Fig 2.7) and this fits well with the notion that force is generated by numerous cross-bridges which are each active over a small distance. In experiments such as these with whole muscles there is likely to be significant series compliance in the tendons and attachments to the apparatus which will complicate the interpretation. However similar observations have been made with small fibre segments where series compliance has been largely eliminated (see Section 2.4.6).

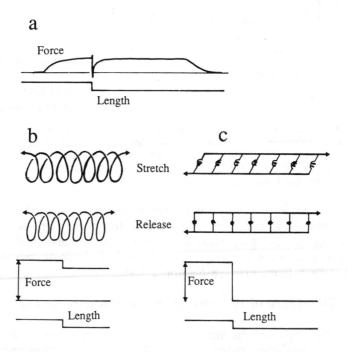

Fig. 2.7 The effect of a rapid short release on muscle force. **a**, release of stimulated frog muscle (Gasser & Hill, 1924). **b**, a short release of a long spring would gives a small reduction in force. **c**, force generated by a number of small short springs acting in parallel; a short release leads to a large drop in force.

The force produced by a muscle is proportional to the cross-sectional area of the muscle rather than its length.

Working outwards from the central Z line of a muscle fibre it can be seen (Fig. 2.8) that the forces exerted by each half-sarcomere on the adjacent Z line are opposed to one another and so do not summate along the length of the fibre. The intermediate sarcomeres serve to form a rigid connection between the two ends and, for the purposes of generating isometric force, could be replaced with a piece of string.

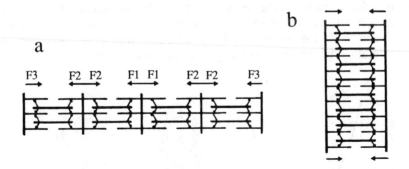

Fig. 2.8 Force generated by sarcomeres in series and in parallel. **a**, sarcomeres in series. The forces F1 and F2 are opposed, leaving only F3 to exert force at the ends of the muscle. **b**, the same number of actin and myosin filaments arranged in parallel to give four times the isometric force of **a**.

Although force is independent of length this is not the case for speed of shortening. At the onset of contraction all sarcomeres in a muscle fibre will begin to shorten more or less at the same time and at the same velocity. If the muscle were only one sarcomere long and shortened from 3 to 2 μm in a tenth of a second then the velocity of shortening would be 10μm per sec. If the muscle consisted of 100 sarcomeres in series the shortening velocity would be 1mm per second and for a muscle an inch long (2.5 cm) containing about 10,000 sarcomeres in series, the velocity of shortening would be 10cm per second. To compare speed of shortening in muscles of different lengths the velocity is often expressed as muscle lengths per second or as sarcomere lengths per second.

Power is the product of force and velocity. Since force is proportional to the cross sectional area of a muscle, and velocity to the length, it follows that power is proportional to the product of these, namely volume. Thus a short fat muscle (Fig. 2.8b) will generate a high force but have a low maximum velocity of shortening, while a long, thin muscle (Fig. 2.8a) will produce little force but shorten rapidly. The muscles will, however, have the same volumes and, therefore, maximum power outputs. Maximum power is usually obtained at about one-third Vmax so that although the maximum power may be the same in the two muscles, the velocity at which this occurs will be different.

2.4 Force-velocity characteristics

The length-tension characteristics of skeletal muscle together with the rapid release experiments established, in broad terms, the type of structure required to explain force generation. Further information about the nature of the myosin-actin interaction has been obtained by consideration of the force-velocity characteristics of muscle.

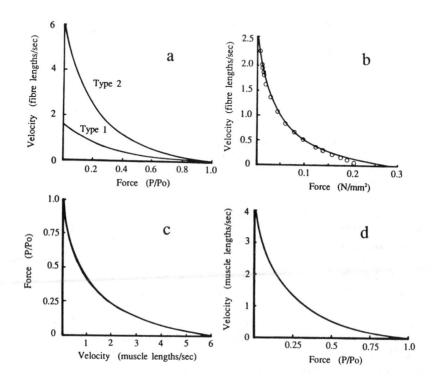

Fig. 2.9 Force-velocity relationships for different muscle preparations. **a**, human type 1 and type 2 fibres estimated from preparations of isolated human muscle obtained at surgery; 37°C. **b**, frog anterior tibialis, 2.7°C, single fibre with measurements made by length clamping. Hill's equation fitted to data less than 80% Po, note the deviation at high forces. **c**, rat medial gastrocnemius, 26°C, using isokinetic releases. **d**, human elbow flexors, values estimated from measurements made *in situ* (Wilkie, 1950).

We have seen that the force generated by a muscle depends on the filament overlap and therefore length, but the force generated also varies with the velocity at which it is shortening or lengthening (Fig. 2.9). Despite increasing experimental sophistication in the way force and velocity are controlled and measured, the basic form of the relationship remains the same as described in the 1920s and 1930s when there was the first great surge of interest in the relationships between force, velocity and energy liberation during contraction.

As the velocity of shortening increases so the force sustained by the muscle rapidly diminishes, eventually reaching a velocity at which force can no longer be sustained at all; this is the maximum velocity of unloaded shortening (Vmax).

The force at zero velocity of shortening (isometric force) is often referred to as Po. Muscles of different sizes and therefore different isometric strengths can be compared by expressing the force (P) at a particular velocity as a fraction of Po.

During an isometric contraction there is no movement, no external work is done by the muscle and all the energy liberated appears in the form of heat. During shortening, heat is still produced but the muscle also performs work which is the product of the force and distance moved. It was first observed by Fenn in 1923 and 1924 that during shortening the total energy liberated, in the form of heat plus work, is greater than that occurring during an isometric contraction (Fenn effect). This observation stimulated a great deal of work and speculation about the nature of the contractile process. In 1938 A.V. Hill reported his observations that both the extra amount of heat liberated and the work done are proportional to the distance shortened in a contraction. If x is the distance shortened then the extra energy liberated is $Px + ax$ or $(P+a)x$, where a is a constant related to heat production. The rate of energy liberation is $(P+a)x/t$, or $(P+a)V$. Hill found that this was proportional to the quantity $(Po-P)$, giving the so called "characteristic" equation:

$$(P + a)V = b(Po - P) \qquad (2.1)$$

This is the equation of a hyperbola in which the axes have been moved by the constants a and b. The equation is a valuable way of describing the characteristics of a muscle and estimating Vmax where this cannot be easily measured. When fitting experimental data a useful linear transformation of Hill's equation is:

$$P/Po = b(Po - P)/V.Po - a/Po$$

Plotting P/Po against (Po - P)/V.Po gives a line with slope b and an intercept a/Po. Vmax can be obtained from equation 2.1 by putting P = 0, so that Vmax = b.Po/a.

The linear form tends, however, to give undue weight to high values of P where there is deviation from Hill's equation. Examples of force-velocity curves for various muscles are given in Fig. 2.9.

Hill's characteristic equation is an empirical description of the experimental data and does not embody any hypothesis about the way in which force is generated. Any explanation of the mechanics of force generation must be able to account for the observed force-velocity characteristics and the way in which energy liberation increases with shortening.

2.4.1 Cross-bridge kinetics

The concept of cross-bridge action and the model of the myosin molecule with a head that rotates and stretches a compliant portion is largely the result of the theories put forward by A.F.Huxley in 1957 and extended by Huxley and Simmons in 1971.

The maximum number of cross-bridges that can be formed will be set by the degree of filament overlap and the number of actin binding sites exposed by the binding of calcium to troponin. However, only a proportion will be attached at any one moment and this fraction will be a function of the rates of attachment and detachment. The rate constant for attachment is usually designated f and that for detachment, g.

If n is the fraction of cross-bridges attached, then the rate of attachment is given by $f(1-n)$ and the rate of detachment by $g \times n$. During a strictly isometric contraction when force has reached a constant value, the rates of attachment and detachment will be equal so

$$f(1-n) = g.n$$

or $n = f/(f+g)$

If the rate constants for attachment and detachment were equal the proportion of attached cross-bridges would be 50%. During an isometric contraction the proportion of attached cross-bridges is usually thought to be about 80% which means that f is about twice g. The proportion of attached cross-bridges, given by the fraction n, is independent of the absolute values of f and g provided that there is sufficient time for the equilibrium between attached and detached cross-bridges to be established; this will only be the case during isometric contractions when the actin and myosin binding sites remain in the same relative positions.

In contractions where the muscle is shortening, the force sustained (P) is less than isometric force (Po) for two reasons. First the average force exerted by each cross-bridge is less than in the isometric state, and second there are fewer cross-bridges attached.

Figure 2.10 shows how the tension sustained in each cross-bridge depends on the extent to which the compliant S2 portion of the myosin is stretched. As the actin filaments move past the myosin filaments during shortening, S2 becomes shorter reducing the tension generated by individual cross-bridges. The faster the movement the greater the shortening of S2 and the less the tension sustained. In some cases the myosin head may not detach in time to prevent it being carried into a position where it is no longer exerting tension but is resisting movement (Fig. 2.10 **b** iii). With higher velocities the proportion of cross-bridges carried into this position increases, and there comes a velocity at which the resistive force generated by compressing cross-bridges equals the force generated by cross-bridges where rotation of the myosin head is stretching the S2 portion. In this situation no net force is generated by the muscle and this velocity is the maximum velocity of shortening (Vmax).

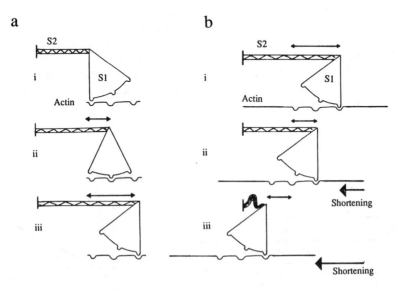

Fig. 2.10 Cross-bridge attachment during isometric and shortening contractions. **a**, isometric state, attachment and rotation of the myosin head (i - iii) causes extension of the compliant S2 portion. **b**, shortening; i, isometric condition, S2 fully extended; ii, slow shortening with the actin filament moving from right to left; the average extension of S2 is less than in **b** (i); iii, rapid shortening with the S2 portion in compression. The double headed arrows indicate the amount of stretch or compression in S2.

If the muscle is shortening and the actin binding sites are moving past the myosin cross-bridges, there will only be a limited time during which attachment can take place. The faster the velocity of shortening, the shorter the time available and the lower the proportion of cross-bridges that will manage to attach in the region over which the cross-bridge can exert a useful force. The number of attached cross-bridges, and therefore the force generated during shortening, will be less than during an isometric contraction.

The mathematical formulation of the 1957 theory allows quantitative predictions of the force-velocity relationship.

2.4.2 *A.F. Huxley's 1957 model*

In this model the myosin binding site oscillates backwards and forwards and, when it attaches to an actin binding site, exerts a force pulling the binding site towards the central equilibrium position (Fig. 2.11a). To produce movement in one direction it is necessary to specify that the attachment will only occur when the myosin binding site is on one side of the equilibrium position; the force generated being proportional to the displacement x. Cross-bridges which are carried beyond the central position will generate force opposing the movement; to keep this opposing force to a minimum it is necessary that there should be a rapid dissociation once the cross-bridge moves into regions where the value of x is negative; the rate constants for attachment (f) and detachment (g) are postulated to vary with displacement as shown in Fig. 2.11b. The rate constant for detachment for negative values of x is assigned a high and constant value (g_2).

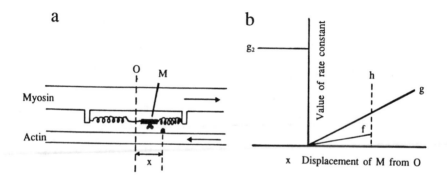

Fig. 2.11 Mechanical model forming the basis of Huxley's 1957 theory. **a**, the myosin binding sites M oscillates about the equilibrium position O and can bind to the actin only for positive values of x. **b**, rate constants for attachment (f) and detachment (g) of myosin to actin. h is the maximum displacement of the myosin head at which binding can occur. For negative values of x, f is zero and g has a high and constant value (g_2).

The linear manner in which the rate constants were chosen to vary with displacement from the equilibrium position is arbitrary but has the advantage that it generates soluble differential equations. Using these equations the proportion of cross-bridges which are attached can be calculated, both as a function of displacement from the equilibrium position and of the velocity at which the actin and myosin filaments slide past one another.

Figure 2.12 shows the distribution of cross-bridges for different types of contraction. During an isometric contraction (**a**) cross-bridges are all in the range 0-h; in (**b**), with slow sliding of the filaments past one another, fewer cross-bridges are attached near to the position h and some have been carried into the region beyond the equilibrium position so that the bridges are compressed and oppose movement. At a high velocity of shortening (**c**) there is little time for cross-bridge attachment so that the total number of attached bridges is reduced and a large proportion of these are carried beyond the equilibrium position and are therefore opposing force generation. The total force generated is proportional to the integral of n.x, that is the number of cross-bridges attached in each position multiplied by their displacement from the equilibrium position since the force in S2 is proportional to the displacement.

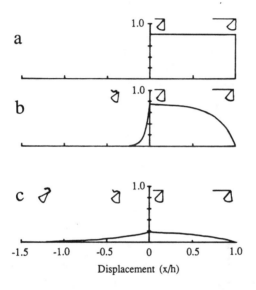

Fig. 2.12   Distribution of cross-bridges calculated from Huxley's 1957 theory. **a**, isometric contraction, **b** & **c** increasing velocities of shortening. Vertical axis, the proportion of available cross-bridges; horizontal axis, displacement of myosin cross-bridge from the equilibrium position in units of h (see Fig. 2.11a).

When the opposing force due to cross-bridges in compression equals the force generated by the cross-bridges in the region 0 - h the net result is no force production by the muscle. The velocity at which this occurs is the maximum velocity of shortening. For a general review of cross-bridge kinetics, see Irving (1987).

2.4.3   *ATP splitting during shortening*

With a judicious selection of rate constants, the Huxley model produces a remarkably good fit of the observed force velocity characteristics for skeletal muscle. It also gives an explanation of the

Fenn effect: if one ATP is hydrolysed with every cross-bridge dissociation, the rate at which heat and work are produced will depend on the rate of cross-bridge turnover. In the isometric state the rate constant for cross-bridge detachment is relatively low but in the region beyond the equilibrium position g_2 is high and therefore turnover and liberation of energy will be high. As the velocity of shortening increases so the number of cross-bridges carried into an orientation where detachment is rapid, also increases, accounting for the increase in production of heat plus work. The rate of energy liberation will, however, begin to level off with increasing velocity since, although turning over more rapidly, there will be fewer cross-bridges actually attached.

2.4.4 *Force during muscle stretch*

In the body muscles work in pairs, while one muscle shortens its antagonist is stretched and many movements, such as walking down stairs or lowering weights, involve the extension of active muscles (Fig. 2.13a).

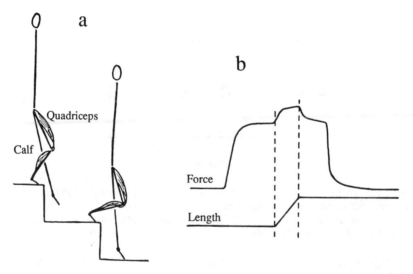

Fig. 2.13 Stretching muscles. **a**, the quadriceps and calf muscles are stretched when lowering the body weight down a step. **b**, mouse soleus muscle stimulated to develop maximum isometric force and then stretched at a constant rate.

The force generated during this type of movement is considerably greater than the isometric force (Fig. 2.13b) and varies with velocity. With increasing velocity of stretch, force begins to plateau, reaching a value of about 1.8 times the isometric force (Fig. 2.14). The increased force can be explained in terms of Huxley's model in that during a stretch the compliant portions S2 of individual cross-bridges are stretched further than is normally the case during isometric contractions (Fig. 2.15a).

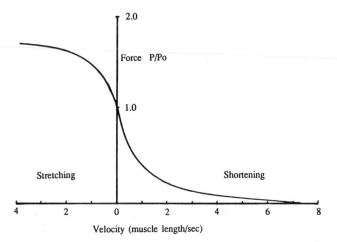

Fig. 2.14 Force of mouse soleus muscle during stretch and shortening; 26°C.

Figure 2.15b shows the distribution of cross-bridges as predicted by Huxley's sliding filament model assuming that the rate constant of detachment (g) continues to increase linearly beyond h. With increasing speed of stretch, the number of cross-bridges attached will decrease but those attached will sustain more force, thus the force maintained by a muscle during stretch tends towards a plateau at higher velocities.

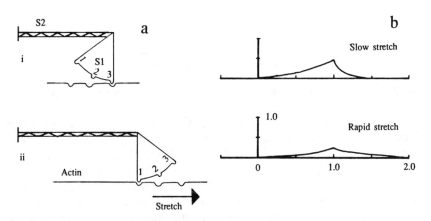

Fig. 2.15 Behaviour of cross-bridges during stretch. **a**, movement of actin from left to right (ii) produces greater stretch of the S2 component than in the isometric condition (i). **b**, distribution of cross-bridges for slow and rapid stretch.

The overall shape of the curve shown in Fig. 2.14 with force increasing with stretch and decreasing with shortening, may have important consequences for the stability of sarcomeres acting in series. If one sarcomeres is stronger than the next, it might be imagined that the stronger would pull out and extend the weaker, eventually to destroy the fibre. However this is not the case since when the sarcomeres begin to move the force generated by the stronger will fall as it shortens (moving down the right hand portion of the curve in Fig. 2.14) while the force of the weaker sarcomere will increase as it is stretched (moving up the left hand side of Fig. 2.14). Consequently sarcomeres of unequal strength (due to differences in length, activation or even damage) can co-exist and function to transmit force along the length of the fibre. This stabilising process may underlie the process of creep (Section 2.2).

2.4.5 *ATP splitting during stretching*

The Huxley model provides a remarkably good explanation for the overall kinetics of cross-bridge behaviour in generating force but it does not explain two important features of muscle function, first the decreased rate of ATP hydrolysis when muscles are stretched and secondly the changes in force during very rapid movements.

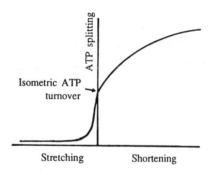

Fig. 2.16 ATP turnover in muscle allowed to shorten or while being stretched.

On the basis of one molecule of ATP split for every cross-bridge detachment, the model predicts that ATP splitting will increase with increasing velocity both of shortening and stretching. However, heat production falls to low values when muscle is stretched, a fact first noticed by Fenn. More recently, Curtin & Davies (1973) showed that ATP splitting was likewise very low during stretching (Fig. 2.16).

To accommodate this observation, the model requires only minor modification, namely the existence of an attached cross-bridge state where detachment does not involve ATP splitting - this could be the back reaction of f. Detachment during shortening would mainly involve ATP splitting but during stretch detachment would be primarily a mechanical process, thus in Fig. 2.15a, dissociation with the myosin head attached in position 3 might require ATP whereas detachment from position 1 would not.

2.4.6 *Rapid transients*

If contracting muscle is shortened very rapidly force falls as the compliant portions S2 are unloaded. According to the Huxley 1957 model these cross-bridges would be expected to detach and re-attach leading to a smooth single phase regeneration of force. The experimental observation, however, of a biphasic process. There is a very rapid initial recovery of force from T_1 to T_2 (Fig. 2.17a) followed by a slower phase during which the force returns to the isometric tension. The explanation proposed by Huxley & Simmons in 1970 is that the rapid phase of force recovery is due to rotation of the heads of the unloaded bridges thereby re-stretching the compliant S1 component (Fig. 2.17b).

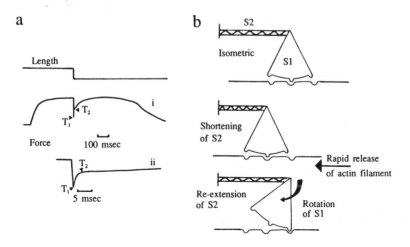

Fig. 2.17 Force transients during rapid release. **a**, force response shown on a slow (i) and fast (ii) time base. **b**, shortening of S2 during rapid release is compensated for by the rapid rotation of the myosin head portion, producing the T_1-T_2 recovery.

The slow phase of force recovery, from T_2 to full isometric force, is ascribed to detachment and reattachment of cross-bridges, so that the conditions of the isometric contraction are re-established. These observations form the basis for the model of a rotating myosin head which has been used throughout this chapter.

The size of the various transients differs with the extent of the rapid release (Fig. 2.18). For small releases the size of the drop from isometric force to T_1 (T_1 curve) is almost linearly related to the size of the release which is consistent with the transition being due to the S2 portion of the myosin molecule acting as a compliance that obeys Hook's law. The T_1-T_2 transition (T_2 curve) shows a plateau for small releases which is thought to correspond to the range of movement over which rotation of the myosin head can fully take up the slack in the S2 portion. For longer releases the rotation can only partially compensate for the change in length of the S2 portion and so T_2 is less than the isometric force.

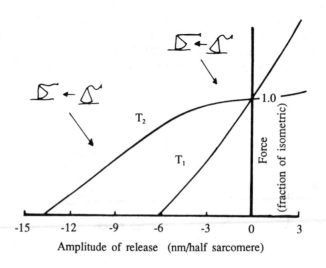

Fig. 2.18 The effect of different length changes on the T_1 and T_2 forces (Fig. 2.17a). Insets show that after long releases rotation of S1 cannot fully compensate for the slack in S2.

2.5 Biochemistry of force generation

In the last 20 years two major preoccupations of muscle biophysics have been to establish whether or not ATP is the immediate source of energy for the generation of force and to determine how the transduction of chemical energy into mechanical events takes place within the muscle.

Although ATP plays such a central role in muscle metabolism this is not immediately obvious from measurements of metabolite levels in contracting muscle. During a sustained contraction there can be large changes in phosphocreatine, breaking down to creatine and inorganic phosphate, together with increases in lactate and hydrogen ion (decrease in pH). ATP, however, changes very little in the course of a contraction (see Chapter 8) and, in 1949, A.V. Hill issued a challenge to biochemists to prove that ATP is the immediate source of energy for muscular contraction. The difficulty in doing so arises because there are a number of reactions, some very rapid, which maintain the level of ATP within the muscle fibre. ADP is rapidly rephosphorylated from phosphocreatine by the enzyme creatine kinase which is abundant in muscle (Fig 2.19) and the equilibrium of the reaction is well over to the side of ATP formation so that the ATP level remains virtually constant until the phosphocreatine has become almost exhausted. It was not until Cain & Davies (1962) used dinitroflurobenzene to inhibit creatine kinase that unequivocal evidence of ATP involvement in contraction was first demonstrated. Glycolysis and oxidative metabolism also act to restore levels of ATP but these processes can be blocked with the inhibitors iodoacetate and cyanide respectively.

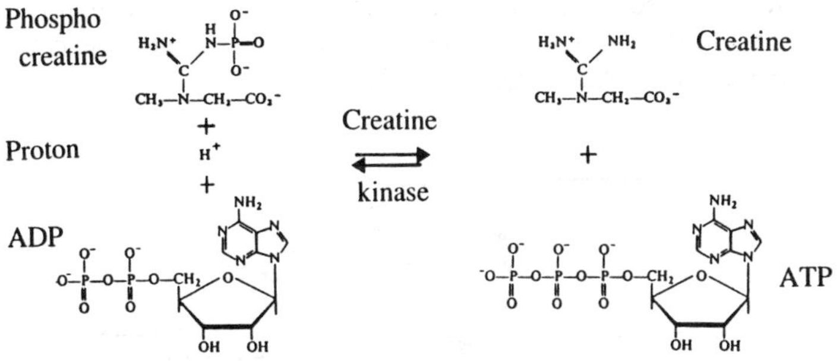

Fig. 2.19 The action of creatine kinase. The phosphorylation of ADP involves the absorption of H^+ and decrease in pH.

There is a natural and continuing interest in the mechanism whereby the energy liberated by hydrolysis of ATP is transformed into mechanical work. There is general agreement that the interaction of actin, myosin and ATP proceeds in a stepwise fashion and that the intermediate stages can, or eventually will, be identified with different mechanical steps in the cross-bridge cycle.

The first indication of the complex nature of the actomyosin ATPase was the observation that on adding actin to a mixture of myosin and ATP, there is an initial rapid appearance of phosphate (phosphate burst) before the system settled down to a steady, and lower, rate of ATP hydrolysis.

The explanation of the phosphate burst is that myosin, which has been preincubated with ATP, has bound to it the hydrolysis products

ADP and Pi.   These products are released when actin and myosin combine.

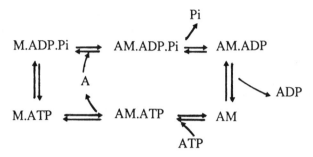

Fig. 2.20 Steps in the hydrolysis of ATP by actin and myosin.

Detailed studies of the kinetics have demonstrated a large number of possible intermediates. The main steps thought to be involved in a normal cross-bridge cycle are shown in Fig. 2.20 and their probable relation to the mechanical events in Fig. 2.21.

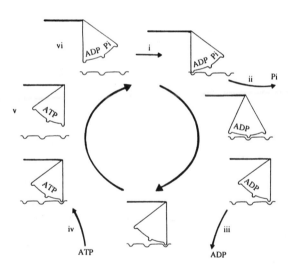

Fig. 2.21 Stages in the cross-bridge cycle corresponding to the different biochemical steps shown in Fig. 2.20. Force is generated between steps ii & iii.

Attachment of actin and myosin (i) is a reversible process which will give stiffness to the muscle (i.e. it will resist if stretched) but does not itself generate force. The release of phosphate from the actomyosin complex (ii) is thought to initiate the changes that result in force generation (rotation of the S1 head in this model). Towards the end of the rotation phase ADP is released (iii) and the actomyosin complex can then bind ATP (iv). Having done so the actin and myosin dissociate with the ATP bound to myosin (v). The bound ATP is then hydrolysed and the products remain bound to the protein (vi); this last process is thought to activate the S1 unit making it ready to bind to actin again. Skinned fibre preparations can be used to investigate the mechanical correlates of the enzymic steps (e.g. Cooke & Pate, 1985). Adding phosphate to contracting skinned fibres decreases the force generated. This is thought to be a result of slowing the rate of release of phosphate (ii) leading to an accumulation of cross-bridges in the state preceding the development of force. Consequently there will be a lower proportion of cross-bridges in a state where they can develop force. The rate of unloaded shortening is determined by the rate of cross-bridge detachment in the region beyond the useful range of movement of the cross-bridge head (g_2, -ve values of x, Fig. 2.12). The detachment is thought to correspond to reaction iv involving the binding of ATP and reaction v, the dissociation step. Phosphate does not influence the rate of reaction iv and therefore does not affect the force-velocity characteristics. ADP, on the other hand, will inhibit reaction iii, the release of ADP, and will thus reduce the proportion of cross-bridges which reach the stage where they can dissociate. This leads to an accumulation of cross-bridges in a force generating state. For an isometric contraction, increased ADP causes a higher force but during shortening a larger proportion of cross-bridges will be carried into a position where they oppose movement (see Fig. 2.10) leading to a reduction in force at a given velocity and in Vmax, the maximum velocity of shortening.

2.6 References and further reading

Astbury, W.T. (1950). X-ray studies of muscle. *Proceedings of the Royal Society B* **137**, 58-63.

Cain, D.F. & Davies, R.E. (1962). Breakdown of adenosine triphosphate during a single contraction of working muscle. *Biochemical and Biophysical Research Communications* **8**, 361-6.

Cooke, R. & Pate, E. (1985). The effects of ADP and phosphate on the contraction of muscle fibres. *Biophysical Journal* **48**, 789-98.

Curtin, N.A. & Davies, R.E. (1973). Chemical and mechanical change during stretching of activated frog skeletal muscle. *Symposia on Quantitative Biology* **XXVII**, 619-26.

Fenn, W.O. (1923). A quantitative comparison between the energy liberated and the work performed by the isolated sartorius muscle of the frog. *Journal of Physiology* **58**, 175-203.

Gasser, H.S & Hill, A.V. (1924). The dynamics of muscular contraction. *Proceedings of the Royal Society B* **96**, 398-437.

Gordon, A.M., Huxley, A.F. & Julian, F.J. (1966). The variation in isometric tension with sarcomere length in vertebrate muscle fibres. *Journal of Physiology* **184**, 170-92.

Hill, A.V. (1938). The heat of shortening and the dynamic constants of muscle *Proceedings of the Royal Society B* **126**, 136-95.

Hill, A.V. (1949). Adenosine triphosphate and muscular contraction. *Nature* **163**, 320.

Huxley, A.F. (1957). Muscle structure and theories of contraction. *Progress in Biophysics and Biophysical Chemistry* **7**, 255-318.

Huxley, A.F. & Peachey, L.D. (1961). The maximum length for contraction in vertebrate striated muscle. *Journal of Physiology* **156**, 150-65.

Huxley, A.F. & Simmons, R.M. (1971). Proposed mechanism of force generation in striated muscle. *Nature* **233**, 533-8.

Huxley, H.E. (1969). The mechanism of muscular contraction. *Science* **164**, 1356-66.

Irving, M. (1987). Muscle mechanics and probes of the crossbridge cycle. In: *Fibrous Protein Structure,* ed. J.M. Squire & P.J. Vibert. London, Academic Press, pp. 495-528.

Ramsey, R.W. & Street, S.F. (1940). The length tension diagram of isolated skeletal muscle fibres of the frog. *Journal of Cellular and Comparative Physiology* **15**, 11-34.

Wilkie, D.R. (1950). The relation between force and velocity in human muscle. *Journal of Physiology* **110**, 249-80.

Woledge, R.C., Curtin, N.A. & Homsher, E. (1985). Energetic aspects of muscle contraction. *Monographs of the Physiological Society* No. **41**. London, Academic Press.

Chapter 3

INNERVATION AND ELECTRICAL ACTIVITY

3.1 Connections between nerve and muscle

3.1.1 *First contacts*

In the human embryo, probably as early as 10 to 11 weeks of gestation, developing motor axons from the spinal cord invade the foetal muscle where they make contact with primary myotubes and, later, with the secondary and tertiary myotubes (for details of the growth and development of muscle, see Chapter 5). At first a number of axons form synapses with each embryonic fibre but as the muscle matures all but one of the synapses are lost (Fig. 3.1). Before innervation the whole membrane surface of the myotube is covered with acetyl choline receptors (AChR) but with the onset of contractile activity these *extra-junctional* receptors are lost and the acetyl choline receptors become restricted to the muscle membrane forming the neuromuscular junction.

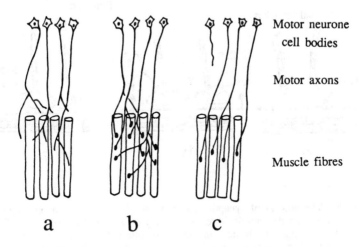

Motor neurone
cell bodies

Motor axons

Muscle fibres

a   b   c

Fig. 3.1 Invasion of muscle by motor nerves. **a**, motor axons branch and invade the foetal muscle. **b**, multiple synapses are formed with each foetal muscle fibre. **c**, mature muscle fibres. Each fibre is now innervated by one motor axon branch.

The loss of receptors is activity dependent and thought to be a consequence of calcium release in the active fibre switching off AChR gene transcription which raises the question of how AChR survives under the neuromuscular junction in the mature fibre (Laufer *et al*, 1989). Several neuropeptides are released together with acetyl choline from the presynaptic nerve terminal and one of these, *calcitonin gene-related peptide*, is thought to cause the expression of the AChR gene in nuclei immediately under the neuromuscular junction. Thus the nuclei which can be seen clustered in the region of the junction (see Fig. 1.18) differ in their gene expression from the majority of nuclei in the fibre.

3.1.2 *Loss of multiple innervation*

How the muscle fibre passes from a state of multiple innervation to one where it is supplied by only one motoneurone is an intriguing question.   With nerve muscle preparations maintained *in vitro* the rejection process can be prevented by addition of inhibitors such as leupeptin which block the action of proteolytic enzymes activated by calcium.   The rejection can also be prevented by reducing the calcium concentration in the extracelluar fluid.   On the other hand, a high concentration of potassium in the surrounding medium has been shown to speed up the detachment of motor axon branches.

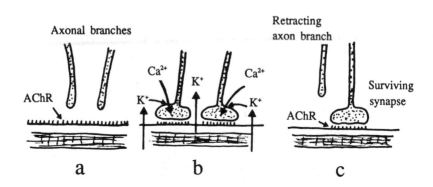

Fig. 3.2   The process of synaptic rejection. **a**, multiple motor axons approach and make contact with the muscle fibre. **b**, activity evoked in the fibre causes K⁺ release and opening of calcium channels in the presynaptic axonal membrane. **c**, the mature muscle fibre. The contractile activity in the muscle fibres has had two effects: (i) it reduces the number of extra-junctional acetyl choline receptors (AChR) and (ii) it causes the rejection of all but one neuromuscular junction.

The loss of multiple innervation appears to be brought about by the contractile activity of the developing fibre which, paradoxically, is the result of stimulation by the same attached nerve endings (Fig. 3.2). Contractile activity of the muscle fibre releases potassium ions into the surrounding extracellular space, activating K^+-dependent calcium channels in the membranes of nearby axon terminations. Calcium enters the nerve terminal, stimulating calcium-dependent proteases which attack the structure of the terminal (probably the neurofilaments), causing the axon to retract. The single surviving axonal attachment may be the one which is largest and most well developed; size may be an advantage since it will give a larger ratio of volume to surface area, keeping the calcium concentration relatively low (Vrbova & Lowrie, 1989). In more mature nerve terminals there might be a change in the number or sensitivity of the K^+-dependent calcium channels. Nerve and muscle therefore have an uneasy coexistence, the nerve striving to innervate muscle fibres while the muscle fibres appear to do their best to reject those axons that make contact.

If a muscle fibre becomes denervated, the whole surface membrane again becomes covered with acetyl choline receptors. Nearby healthy axons are stimulated to sprout and branch. Trophic substances might be released from the denervated fibre to stimulate axonal growth, but the sprouting could also be a permissive process. Active muscle may suppress axonal branching in the same way as it causes the retraction of redundant synapses and only when the fibre is quiescent might sprouting begin. Several adjacent axons may be induced to sprout and make contact with the denervated fibre, and the process of multiple innervation followed by rejection will occur as first took place in the foetal muscle.

3.2 The motor unit

In a mature muscle one motoneurone will, through its axonal branches, supply a number of fibres scattered throughout the muscle. In a healthy muscle the innervation is almost entirely random and adjacent fibres are most likely to be supplied by branches from different motoneurones (Fig. 3.3). All the muscle fibres supplied by one motoneurone form a *motor unit*. If a motoneurone fires, all the muscle fibres in that unit will contract at the same time, producing a synchronous electrical discharge (action potential) and generation of force (twitch). The size of the action potential, recorded from the surface of the muscle, and the size of the twitch, will be proportional to the number of fibres within the contracting motor unit. Within a single muscle there is a range of motor unit size, the number and type of fibres in each depending on the function of the motoneurone. The fast motoneurones support large motor units while slow motoneurones support small units (see Chapter 4, section 4.5).

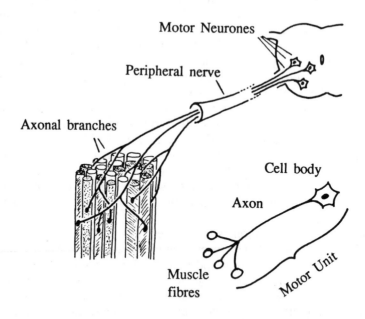

Fig. 3.3 The concept of the motor unit. A motor unit consists of the motoneurone and all the scattered muscle fibres which it innervates.

The number of fibres constituting a motor unit varies from muscle to muscle and may be as few as 10 fibres in a small hand muscle to several thousand in a large muscle such as the quadriceps. The number of fibres depends not only on the size of the muscle but also on its function. The finer the control of movement required, the smaller will be the size of the motor units.

3.3 The neuromuscular junction

A neuromuscular junction is the synaptic connection at which the axon branch of the motoneurone meets the muscle fibre. At this point the membranes of the muscle and nerve are closely opposed to one another with the sarcolemma thrown into elaborate folds (see Fig. 1.18). In the presynaptic terminal acetyl choline (ACh) is stored in vesicles, together with ATP and possibly one or more peptide hormones (see Section 3.1.1). Action potentials which originate in the motoneurone arrive at the axon termination and allow an influx of calcium through voltage-sensitive channels. The increased intracellular calcium causes the ACh-containing vesicles to fuse with the presynaptic nerve membrane and release their contents into the synaptic cleft. The release is, therefore, dependent on the presence of external calcium and is depressed by high magnesium concentrations (Katz, 1966; Jones 1987). The amount of ACh released from a single synaptic vesicle is referred to as a quantum.

In conditions where there is a low plasma ionised-calcium such as hypoparathyroidism, severe rickets or during respiratory alkalosis caused by overbreathing, a condition known as tetany can develop. This is an involuntary contraction, often of the facial muscles, the hand or calf (*carpopedal spasm*). The low plasma ionised calcium leads to an increased excitability of motoneurones causing them to discharge inappropriately.

The post synaptic muscle fibre membrane contains acetyl choline receptors (AChR) which are situated mainly at the crests of the folds (Salpeter, 1987). Cholinesterase, which hydrolytses acetyl choline, is synthesised by the muscle fibre and is secreted into the synaptic cleft where it binds to the extracellular matrix (mostly the basement membrane of the muscle) which fills the cleft (Rotundo, 1987).

3.3.1 *End plate potentials*

Binding of ACh to the post-synaptic receptor causes a depolarisation of the muscle fibre membrane. The extent of the depolarisation depends on the number of receptors binding ACh which in turn depends on the number of synaptic vesicles that have discharged into the synaptic cleft.

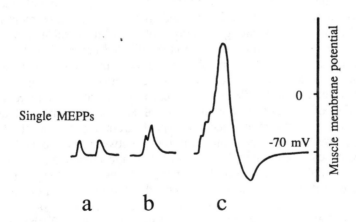

Fig. 3.4 Generation of an action potential at the neuromuscular junction. **a**, miniature end plate potentials (MEPPs). **b**, summation of two quanta but not sufficient to initiate an action potential. **c**, summation of sufficient MEPPs to initiate an action potential.

A single quantum of ACh produces a depolarisation of the muscle membrane known as a *miniature end plate potential* (MEPP). If sufficient quanta of ACh are released at the same time the MEPPs will summate and produce a large enough depolarisation of the muscle membrane to initiate an action potential (Fig. 3.4).

The drug *curare* binds to the ACh receptors acting as a competitive inhibitor preventing depolarization and causing paralysis similar to that seen in *myasthenia gravis* (see Chapter 11, section 11.6). Cholinesterase inactivates ACh by hydrolysis, a process which is inhibited by drugs such as *eserine* and *neostigmine*. These drugs potentiate neuromuscular junction transmission by prolonging the lifetime of ACh within the synaptic cleft and thus increase the chance of binding to an ACh receptor and depolarising the muscle membrane. Free choline is transported back into the presynaptic axon and is resynthesised into ACh within the nerve. This transport can be blocked with *hemicholium* which will produce a myasthenic-like syndrome as the ACh stored in the presynaptic terminal becomes exhausted with continued activity.

Anticholinesterases are used as an antidote to curare and some of the nerve gas poisons and in the management of myasthenia. *Suxamethonium* is a muscle relaxant which acts by binding to ACh receptors and is commonly used during surgery. Unlike curare, suxamethonium causes the postsynaptic membrane to become depolarised so that it passes into an inexcitable refractory state.

3.3.2 *Propagation of the action potential*

When the post-synaptic membrane is sufficiently depolarised a regenerative action potential is initiated in the muscle fibre membrane and will then propagate along the length of the fibre in substantially the same way as propagation occurs in non-myelinated nerve. The T tubular membranes are an extension of the surface membrane and action potentials pass down the T tubules into the interior of the muscle fibre (see Gonzalez-Serratos, 1983). With each action potential there is an inward flux of Na^+ and an outward flux of K^+ into the lumen of the T tubules and the limited extracellular space around each muscle fibre. There is, however, an important difference between muscle and nerve because muscle membranes have a high chloride conductance. As the action potential spreads into the interior of the fibre the T tubular membrane is depolarised at a time when the surface membrane will be repolarising. Potassium accumulating in the T tubule as a result of outward movement during the action potential and slow diffusion and re-uptake gives rise to a significant depolarisation, leading to a prolonged after potential. Consequently a voltage gradient, which could trigger another action potential in the surface membrane, develops between the T tubular membrane in the interior of the fibre and the sarcolemma on the surface of the fibre. The high chloride conductance short circuits this voltage gradient and so prevents repetitive firing (Adrian & Marshall, 1976). In some situations the chloride conductance is reduced (e.g. *myotonia congenita;* see Section 11.10) leading to repetitive firing and slow relaxation of muscle (Adrian & Bryant, 1974).

3.4 Excitation-contraction coupling

As the wave of depolarisation passes down the T tubules there is some interaction with the sarcoplasmic reticulum which results in the release of calcium. The portions of the sarcoplasmic reticulum close to the T tubular membrane are known as the *terminal cisternae,* and it is here that most of the intracellular calcium is stored (Fig. 3.5). It is also from this region that calcium is released in response to depolarisation of the T tubular membrane, forming a crucial link in the chain of events leading from electrical activity in the surface membrane to the interaction of the actin and myosin filaments. The amount of calcium released in response to a single action potential may vary. Some substances will potentiate the twitch (caffeine, Zn, thiocyanate: see Caputo, 1983) while others depress it (dantrolene). Such a change in the force generated by a single action potential is often referred to as a change in excitation-contraction (EC) coupling.

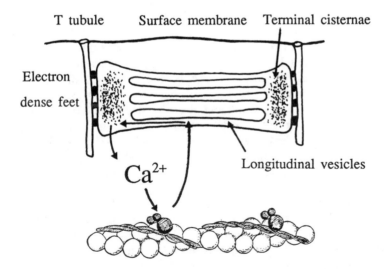

Fig. 3.5 Diagrammatic representation of the arrangement of sarcoplasmic reticulum and T tubules. Calcium is stored and released from the terminal cisternae, interacts with troponin C and is then reaccumulated in the longitudinal vesicles of the SR.

3.4.1   *Calcium release from the sarcoplasmic reticulum*

This stage in the sequence of events leading from excitation to contraction is of critical importance, but the mechanism involved has been, until recently, one of the least well understood aspects of muscle physiology.

There are a number of ways in which calcium might be released from the sarcoplasmic reticulum.

3.4.1.1   *Depolarisation*   One possibility is that the interior of the sarcoplasmic reticulum is polarised with respect to the sarcoplasm and can be depolarised by membrane currents caused by the action potential passing along the T tubule membrane.   Depolarisation of the sarcoplasmic reticulum membrane could then open calcium channels allowing calcium to pass into the interior of the muscle fibre.   If this were the case some counter-movement of cations would be expected. The ionic content of sarcoplasmic reticulum has been examined, using X-ray probe analysis, before and after calcium release, and no evidence has been found of the change in ionic content that would be expected if depolarisation were a crucial step in the process of activation.

3.4.1.2   *Calcium-induced calcium release*   Isolated sarcoplasmic reticulum can be loaded with calcium which is retained against large concentration gradients.   However this calcium is released in response to an increase in calcium concentration on the outside of the sarcoplasmic reticulum membrane.   Thus a small amount of calcium entering the cell during an action potential could act as a trigger causing the release of calcium stored in the sarcoplasmic reticulum (Endo, 1977). In cardiac muscle a large portion of the inward current of the action potential is carried by calcium, one of the functions of which is to trigger further calcium release from intracellular stores in the sarcoplasmic reticulum.   Cardiac muscle is dependent on extracellular calcium for contraction but skeletal muscle can continue to contract for an appreciable time even when external calcium is reduced to a low level.   It is therefore unlikely that calcium entry from the extracelluar space plays a major role in the activation of skeletal muscle.

3.4.1.3   *Movement of voltage sensors*   Skeletal muscle membranes contain a high density of voltage-sensitive calcium channels, identified by the binding of dihydropyridine (DHP), despite the fact that inward calcium fluxes seem to play little or no part in the process of activation. This raises the possibility that the DHP binding sites may no longer function primarily as calcium channels but could have a specialist role as voltage sensors linked to the release of calcium from the sarcoplasmic reticulum (Chandler *et al*, 1976 a,b; Caswell & Brandt, 1989).

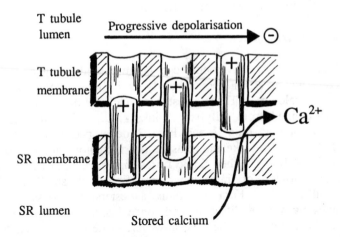

T tubule lumen

Progressive depolarisation $\ominus$

T tubule membrane

Ca^{2+}

SR membrane

SR lumen

Stored calcium

Fig. 3.6. Possible mechanism for the release of calcium. Voltage sensors in the T tubular membrane move outwards in response to depolarisation. With sufficient depolarisation the calcium channels in the sarcoplasmic reticulum membrane are open and calcium escapes into the cytoplasm and diffuses to the myofibrils.

The voltage sensors might be directly linked to calcium channels in the sarcoplasmic reticulum membrane. When the T tubular membrane is sufficiently depolarised the voltage sensor moves into a position that opens the calcium channel, allowing calcium to diffuse from the lumen of the sarcoplasmic reticulum to the interior of the fibre. This calcium may be the total required for activation or a trigger for further calcium-induced calcium release.

The electron dense feet, which can be seen on EM photographs lying between the T tubule and sarcoplasmic reticulum membranes (Fig. 3.5), are almost certainly involved in calcium regulation in skeletal muscle. It is tempting to speculate that they may contain, or even be, the physical link between the voltage sensors in the surface membrane and the calcium channels in the sarcoplasmic reticulum.

3.4.1.4 *Inositol triphosphate* In a large number of tissues calcium is thought to be released as a consequence of the hydrolysis of phosphatidyl inositol; the inositol 1,4,5 triphosphate ($InsP_3$) formed being able to release calcium from internal stores. The voltage sensors might therefore activate a phospholipase and the $InsP_3$ act as a second messenger releasing calcium from the sarcoplasmic reticulum. Although $InsP_3$ can release calcium from the sarcoplasmic reticulum it appears to be too little and too slow to account for the rapid release of calcium in skeletal muscle (Walker *et al*, 1987). $InsP_3$ may well have a role in smooth muscle where calcium release is relatively slow and occurs in response to neurotransmitters and hormones.

3.5 Calcium transients

Intracellular calcium movements can be measured using a number of compounds which either spontaneously emit light or fluoresce in the presence of calcium.   These substances include the protein aequorin which is obtained from jellyfish (Blinks *et al*, 1978) and fluorescent compounds such as quin 2 and Fura 2 developed from the calcium buffer EDTA.   With skeletal muscle the indicators are microinjected into individual fibres, either single fibres that have been dissected from amphibian muscles or into superficial fibres of small bundles of mammalian muscle.   Fura and quin, as esters, can pass across cell membranes by simple diffusion and, once inside, are then hydrolysed to the useful indicator.   There is, however, some concern that the ester may also diffuse into the sarcoplasmic reticulum.

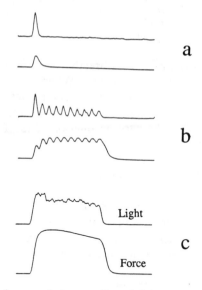

Fig. 3.7   Calcium release and force.   Superficial fibres of a mouse diaphragm preparation were injected with aequorin.   The light signal gives an indication of the intracellular free calcium concentration. **a**, single twitch. **b**, stimulated at 20Hz, and **c**, at 80Hz. The upper trace is the light signal, the lower trace the force.

The stoichiometry and kinetics of calcium binding to the indicators is complex but, to a first approximation, the light signal gives an indication of the magnitude and time course of calcium release (Fig. 3.7).   The calcium released from the sarcoplasmic reticulum diffuses the short distance to the myofibrils where it binds to troponin C on the thin filaments.

3.6 Regulatory proteins

The interaction of actin and myosin in mammalian skeletal muscle is regulated by tropomyosin and the troponin complex. The generally accepted mechanism for this regulation is the "steric blocking" model. At rest the tropomyosin is positioned by troponin so that it covers the myosin binding sites on the actin monomers preventing the formation of cross-bridges. At a critical calcium concentration the troponin changes its conformation, moving the tropomyosin so that the binding sites are exposed, cross-bridges are formed and force develops. Since the troponin spans seven actin monomers, one troponin complex is responsible for controlling the activity of all seven subunits.

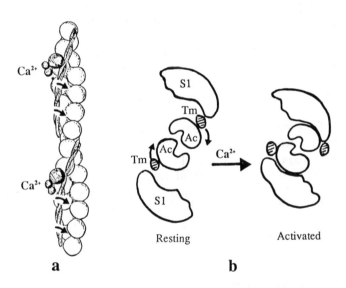

Fig. 3.8 The regulation of actin and myosin interaction. **a**, arrows show the movement of tropomyosin when calcium is bound to troponin. **b**, cross-section of the filament showing how the movement of tropomyosin allows binding of the myosin head to actin. S1, myosin head; Tm, tropomyosin; Ac, actin.

The steric blocking model makes a number of assumptions concerning the shape of the actin filament and the location of the myosin binding sites in relation to the position of tropomyosin (Cohen & Vibert, 1987) and it is possible that the regulation is by a more subtle interaction of actin, myosin and tropomyosin. However the work of Kress *et al* (1986) indicates that tropomyosin movement is an early event in activation, preceeding myosin binding and the generation of force, as would be expected if the regulation was by a mechanical blocking of the binding sites.

3.7 Removal of calcium from the interior of a muscle fibre

Calcium is pumped back into the sarcoplasmic reticulum by a mechanism that requires ATP. The sarcoplasmic reticulum has a very high affinity for calcium and can reduce the intracellular calcium concentration to around 10^{-8} M (Martonosi & Beeler, 1983) and in so doing removes calcium from troponin leading to relaxation.

In cardiac muscle calcium uptake can be enhanced by phosphorylation of the protein *phospholamban*. This phosphorylation is cAMP dependent and may mediate the inotropic effect of catecholamines. This mechanism could account for the speeding up of the relaxation phase reported to occur as a result of noradrenaline action on slow muscle.

Calcium is accumulated in the central portions of the sarcoplasmic reticulum (longitudinal vesicles) and then moves to the terminal cisternae where it is stored. The protein *calsequestrin* helps to bind the calcium here. The internal calcium concentration is around 1mM in the terminal cisternae.

Actively respiring mitochondria will accumulate calcium ions but it is not known whether this accumulation plays a significant role in causing relaxation in normal muscle.

In amphibian and fast mammalian muscles there is a high concentration of the protein *pavalbumin*. This is another calcium binding protein and may have a role in buffering the internal pCa or speeding relaxation, acting in parallel with the sarcoplasmic reticulum to remove calcium from troponin C.

3.8 References and further reading

Adrian, R.H. & Bryant, S.H. (1974). On the repetitive discharge in myotonic muscle fibres. *Journal of Physiology* **240**, 505-15.

Adrian, R.H. & Marshall, M.W. (1976). Action potentials reconstructed in normal and myotonic muscle fibres. *Journal of Physiology* **258**, 125-43.

Blinks, J.R., Rudel, R. & Taylor, S.R. (1978). Calcium transients in isolated amphibian skeletal muscle fibres: detection with aequorin. *Journal of Physiology* **277**, 291-323.

Caputo, C. (1983). Pharmacological investigations of excitation-contraction coupling. In: *Handbook of Physiology, Section 10: Skeletal Muscle*, ed. L.D. Peachey, R.H. Adrian & S.R. Geiger. Bethesda, American Physiological Society, pp. 381-415.

Caswell, A.H. & Brandt, N.R. (1989). Does muscle activation occur by direct mechanical coupling of transverse tubules to sarcoplasmic reticulum? *Trends in Biochemical Sciences* **14**, 161-5.

Chandler, W.K., Rakowski, R.F. & Schneider, M.F. (1976a). Non linear voltage dependent charge movement in frog skeletal muscle. *Journal of Physiology* **254**, 245-83.

Chandler, W.K., Rakowski, R.F. & Schneider, M.F. (1976b). Effects of glycerol treatment and maintained depolarization on charge movement in skeletal muscle. *Journal of Physiology* **254**, 285-316.

Cohen, C. & Vibert, P.J. (1987). Actin filament: images and models. In: *Fibrous Protein Structure*, ed. J.M. Squire & P.J. Vibert. London, Academic Press. pp. 284-306.

Endo, M. (1977). Calcium release from the sarcoplasmic reticulum. *Physiological Reviews* **57**, 71-108.

Gonzalez-Serratos, H. (1983). Inward spread of activation in twitch skeletal muscle fibres. In: *Handbook of Physiology, Section 10: Skeletal Muscle*, ed. L.D. Peachey, R.H. Adrian & S.R. Geiger. Bethesda, American Physiological Society, pp. 325-353.

Jones, S.W. (1987). Presynaptic mechanisms at vertebrate neuromuscular junctions. In: *The Vertebrate Neuromuscular Junction: Neurology and Neurobiology*, Vol. **23**, ed. M.M. Salpeter. New York, Alan R. Liss, Inc., pp. 187-245.

Katz, B. (1966). *Nerve, Muscle, and Synapse*. New York, McGraw-Hill.

Kress, M., Huxley, H.E. & Faruqi, A.R. (1986). Structural changes during activation of frog muscle studied by time-resolved X-ray diffraction. *Journal of Molecular Biology* **188**, 325-42.

Laufer, R., Fontaine, B., Klarsfield, A., Cartaud, J. & Changeux, J.P. (1989). Regulation of acetylcholine receptor biosynthesis during motor endplate morphogenesis. *News in Physiological Sciences* **4**, 5-9.

Martonosi, A.N. & Beeler, T.J. (1983). Mechanism of Ca^{2+} uptake by sarcoplasmic reticulum. In: *Handbook of Physiology, Section 10: Skeletal Muscle*, ed. L.D. Peachey, R.H. Adrian & S.R. Geiger. Bethesda, American Physiological Society, pp. 417-485.

Rotundo, R.L. (1987). Biogenesis and regulation of acetylcholinesterase. In: *The Vertebrate Neuromuscular Junction: Neurology and Neurobiology*, Vol. **23**, ed. M.M. Salpeter. New York, Alan R. Liss, Inc., pp. 247-284.

Salpeter, M.M. (1987).   Vertebrate neuromuscular junctions: general morphology, molecular organization, and functional consequences.   In: *The Vertebrate Neuromuscular Junction: Neurology and Neurobiology*, Vol. **23**, ed. M.M. Salpeter. New York, Alan R. Liss, Inc., pp. 1-54.

Vrbova, G. & Lowrie, M. (1989).   Role of activity in developing synapses, search for molecular mechanisms. *News in Physiological Sciences* **4**, 75-8.

Walker, J.W., Somolyo, A.V., Goldman, Y.E., Somolyo, A.P. & Trentham, D.R. (1987). Kinetics of smooth and skeletal muscle activation by laser pulse photolysis of caged inositol 1,4,5 triphosphate. *Nature* **327**, 249-52.

Chapter 4

HISTOCHEMISTRY, CONTRACTILE PROPERTIES AND MOTOR CONTROL

As early as the seventeenth century a number of authors had commented on the fact that muscles differ in their appearance but it was not until 1873 that the French physician and physiologist Ranvier recognised that skeletal muscles not only differ in colour, some being dark red, others almost white, but that they also have different contractile properties. For example, the soleus muscle at the back of the lower leg is red in appearance and is slow as far as its contractile properties are concerned, while the extensor digitorum longus, a white muscle at the front of the leg, contracts and relaxes rapidly.

4.1 **Histochemistry**

Microscopic differences between muscle fibres can be demonstrated using a variety of histochemical staining reactions on thin sections of frozen, unfixed material. The main stains used to classify skeletal muscle fibres are:

4.1.1 *Myosin ATPase*

The procedure to identify the different types of myosin ATPase in muscle needs to be described in two parts. The first stage consists of incubating the section at either an alkaline or acid pH. Although the values vary somewhat from species to species, in general, fast myosins are inactivated at acid pH (about pH 4.3 to 4.6) while slow myosins are inactivated at alkaline pH (around pH 9.4). Having preincubated the section and inactivated the ATPase activity in one set of fibres, the remaining activity can be visualised by incubating the section with ATP and an excess of calcium at a slightly alkaline pH. The inorganic phosphate liberated precipitates as calcium phosphate. The section is then placed in a solution of cobalt chloride and the calcium in the calcium phosphate precipitate is replaced by cobalt giving cobalt phosphate. Finally the section is washed in ammonium sulphide and the phosphate is replaced leaving a brownish-black precipitate of cobalt sulphide marking the sites of myosin ATPase activity in the muscle fibres. Myosin ATPase is widely used to identify various fibre types, these often being referred to as being of "high" or "low" activity. It is important to remember, however, that the ATPase staining tells nothing of the *level* of myosin ATPase activity at physiological pH, it gives information only about the *stability* of the myosin activity at the pH used for the first step.

4.1.2 *Mitochondrial enzyme activities*

Stains for mitochondrial activity require a substrate that is oxidised and an electron acceptor that is reduced by one of the components of the electron transport chain. A commonly used combination is NADH as substrate and tetrazolium blue as the electron acceptor. The flavoprotein enzyme system (Complex I) that reduces tetrazolium blue is termed NADH tetrazolium reductase. Reduction of the tetrazolium salt gives a blue precipitate. Using succinate as substrate with tetrazolium blue gives a measure of Complex II activity (succinate dehydrogenase).

4.1.3 *Glycolytic activity*

It is possible to visualise a number of enzyme activities as indicators of glycolysis (lactate dehydrogenase, phosphofructokinase, pyruvate kinase). One commonly measured enzyme is myophosphorylase. For this activity the normal process of splitting the 1,4 glycosyl links is driven backwards. Glucose-1-P and small 1-4 glycosyl units are provided in the reaction mixture from which the enzyme forms a long glucose polymer with 1,4 glycosyl links. The polymer can be stained with iodine; four to six glycosyl units produce no colour after which there is a gradation through red and violet to blue-black which is seen when the polymer reaches 30 to 35 units.

Using these three stains the majority of adult mammalian skeletal muscle fibres can be placed in one of three categories, type 1, type 2a or type 2b (Fig. 4.1 and Table 4.1). A fourth fibre subgroup (type 2c) represents myosin found largely in the developing embryo and in regenerating fibres. Increasingly, the histochemical stains are being replaced, or at least complemented, by immunological methods such as using monoclonal antibodies raised against fast or slow myosins.

The soleus muscle in mice and rats is composed almost entirely of type 1 fibres while the extensor digitorum longus consists mainly of type 2a and 2b fibres. This is true of these two muscles in nearly all mammals but most other skeletal muscles contain mixtures of fibre types. Chicken breast muscle contains almost exclusively type 2 fibres but this is not true for other birds, such as the pigeon, that use these muscles for prolonged flight and consequently have a high proportion of oxidative fibres. The high content of myoglobin and cytochrome C in the slow muscle accounts for their red colour.

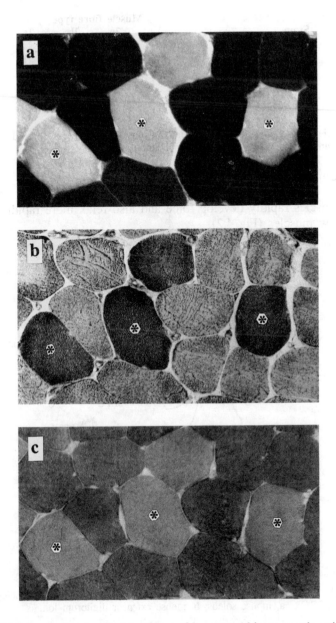

Fig. 4.1 Histochemical stains: Serial sections of human quadriceps muscle stained for a, myosin ATPase, pH 9.4; b, Mitochondrial enzyme activity (NADH tetrazolium reductase); c, glycolytic enzyme activity (phosphorylase). Note the same three type 1 fibres marked (*) in each section.

Stain	Muscle fibre type			
	1	**2a**	**2b**	**2c**
ATPase (pH 9.4)	1+	3+	3+	3+
ATPase (pH 4.6)	3+	0	3+	3+
ATPase (pH 4.3)	3+	0	0	2+
NADH-TR	3+	2+	1+	2+
Phosphorylase	1+	3+	3+	3+

Table 4.1 Histochemical staining of human muscle fibre types. NADH-TR; NADH tetrazolium reductase is a stain for mitochondrial activity.

4.2 Contractile properties

Fast muscles rapidly develop force and also relax more rapidly than do the slow muscles (Fig 4.2).

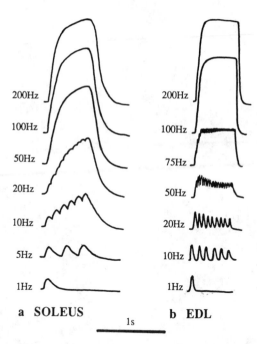

Fig. 4.2 Force generated during a 500msec tetanus at different frequencies (isolated muscles, 25°C). **a**, mouse soleus; **b**, mouse extensor digitorum longus.

The fast extensor digitorum longus muscle, when stimulated at a frequency of 10 to 20Hz, reacts quickly enough for the tension to fall back to the baseline before the next impulse, but in the slower soleus muscle the next impulse comes before relaxation is complete and the contraction is superimposed on the tension remaining from the previous stimulus. In this way the individual twitches are said to summate or fuse. When stimulated at a sufficiently high frequency the muscle will produce a smooth plateau of force. The frequency required to achieve this plateau is known as the fusion frequency and this frequency is higher for fast as compared to slow muscles (Fig. 4.3).

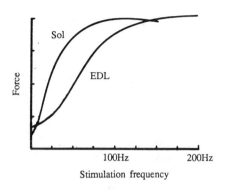

Fig. 4.3 The relationship between force and stimulation frequency. Isolated mouse soleus (Sol) and extensor digitorum longus (EDL), 25°C.

In mammalian muscles the twitch tension is usually about one-fifth to one-tenth of the maximum tetanic force and in this respect differs from amphibian muscle where the twitch tension is around 80% of the maximum force indicating that the muscle is almost fully activated during a twitch. The relatively small twitch of mammalian muscle is presumed to be due to insufficient calcium being released to occupy all the troponin binding sites in response to a single action potential.

There are a number of features that distinguish the contractile properties of fast and slow muscles.

1. *The shape of the twitch.* As shown in Fig. 4.2, the twitch of a fast muscle has an earlier peak and more rapid relaxation than that of a slow muscle. Measurements of contraction time and half relaxation time are commonly made.

2. *Relaxation from an isometric tetanus.* Fig. 4.2 shows the relaxation phase from a tetanus. The last half of the curve approximates a single exponential and a useful measure of speed is the half time of this portion.

3. *Fusion frequency*; this is higher in fast muscles (Fig. 4.3).

4. *Fatiguability.* Muscles vary widely in their response to prolonged activity. Figure 4.4 shows the response of a fast and slow muscle to repetitive stimulation.

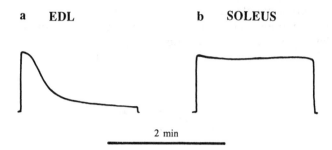

a   **EDL**   b   **SOLEUS**

2 min

Fig. 4.4   Fatigue of fast and slow muscles. Isolated mouse muscles stimulated at 100Hz for 0.25s every second; 25°C. The tracings shows the envelope of the force produced by each contraction.

As first recorded by Ranvier, there is a clear connection between the appearance and contractile properties of certain skeletal muscles such as the red and white muscles of a chicken or the soleus and extensor digitorum longus in a mouse. These muscles are, however, somewhat unusual in consisting predominantly of one fibre type while the majority of skeletal muscles are a mixture of different types. It is important to know whether the different fibre types within a single muscle also have differing contractile properties.

4.3   The relationship between histochemistry and contractile properties

A technique which has been used to investigate this question in rat and cat muscles is illustrated in Fig. 4.5 (Burke *et al*, 1971; Kugelberg, 1973).

By stimulating a single axon or a single motoneurone all the fibres in a one motor unit can be made to contract simultaneously and by using sensitive force recording techniques the contractile characteristics of this motor unit can be determined. The maximum tetanic force generated by the motor unit gives an indication of the number of fibres of which it is composed.

Having measured the size and contractile characteristics of the unit it is necessary to determine the histochemical properties of the muscle fibres of which it is composed. What is required is some way of identifying which fibres within the muscle have been contracting and this is done by stimulating the unit repetitively to deplete the fibres of glycogen. The muscle is then removed, frozen, sectioned and stained for glycogen when the depleted fibres of the motor unit will stand out as pale staining cells against the dark background of undepleted fibres.

Serial sections stained for myosin ATPase, mitochondrial and glycolytic enzymes will define the histochemical properties of the depleted fibres and in this way it is possible to relate the histochemical and contractile properties.

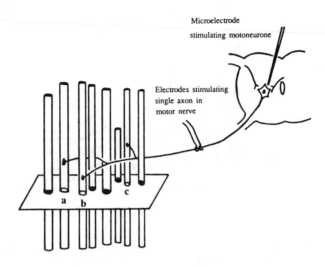

Fig. 4.5 Identification of fibres belonging to a single motor unit. Staining a section shows the fibres that have been depleted of glycogen (**a**, **b** & **c**).

On the basis of size, speed and fatiguability, motor units are found to fall between two extremes, large, fast and fatiguable or small slow and fatigue resistant (Fig. 4.6).

Examining their histochemical properties, the large units tend to be made up of type 2b fibres while the small slow units are predominantly composed of type 1 fibres. Type 2a motor units span a range of size and fatigue resistance which is reflected in the broad spectrum of their mitochondrial enzyme activities. Commonly used nomenclatures which combine information about contractile and histochemical properties are given in Table 4.2, although it should be realised that most classifications oversimplify the situation. Although mammalian skeletal muscles all show similar varieties of fibres when classified by their histochemical properties, there are considerable differences between species as regards contractile characteristics. Thus a slow mouse muscle is still faster than the fastest human skeletal muscle. To some degree this is also true of fibres from different muscles in the same animal, type 1 fibres in the soleus muscle being slower than type 1 fibres in other skeletal muscles.

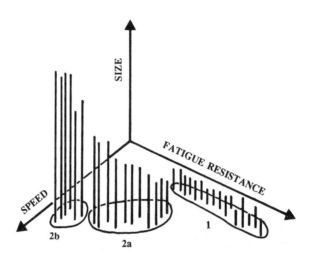

Fig. 4.6 Contractile properties of motor units. The size, speed and fatigue resistance of different types of motor unit, as defined by their histochemical properties.

	G. pig & rabbit	**Cat**
Type 1	SO	S
	Slow twitch,	Slow twitch
	Oxidative	
Type 2a	FOG	FR
	Fast twitch	Fast twitch
	Oxidative/Glycolytic	Fatigue resistant
Type 2b	FG	FF
	Fast twitch	Fast twitch
	Glycolytic	Fatiguable

Table 4.2 The relationships between histochemical fibre type classification and physiological properties. Two ways are given of classifying the physiological properties (Peter *et al*, 1972; Burke *et al*, 1971).

Much of muscle physiology is based on amphibian muscles and these also have a variety of fibre types; unfortunately the system of classification is the opposite of that used with mammalian muscle. Fast frog muscle fibres are type 1 while the slow variety are type 2.

4.3.1 *Characteristics of human muscle fibres*
The technique of inserting microelectrodes into motoneurones or of

dissecting single axons from motor nerves is not well tolerated by human subjects and consequently the relationship between histochemistry and contractile properties is less well established for human muscle fibres. Stephens and co-workers (Garnett *et al*, 1979) stimulated small intramuscular branches of a motor nerve which they believed to be innervating single motor units in human muscle. After characterising the contractile properties and depleting the unit of glycogen by repetitive stimulation, they biopsied the region of the muscle where the unit was thought to be located and used histochemical stains to characterise the fibres. Their results indicate that human fibre types have the same general relationship between contractile properties and histochemical staining as found in other mammalian species.

4.4 The control of fibre type expression

So far we have seen that muscle fibres fall into groups distinguished by their biochemical and physiological properties. Since it is these properties that determine the use that can be made of a muscle it is of prime importance to understand how the expression of genes determining the fibre types is controlled.

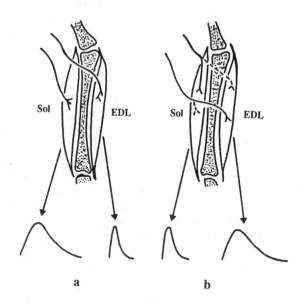

Fig. 4.7 The effect of cross innervation on contractile properties. **a**, before operation with the slow soleus and fast extensor digitorum longus. **b**, after cross innervation; lower traces show the twitch response of the muscles.

The first clue came almost by accident in a series of experiments by Buller *et al* (1960) who were interested in the adaptability of the central nervous system. A motor nerve was transplanted from a muscle situated at the back of an animal's leg to a muscle at the front to see how well the central nervous system could cope with the situation. The results were disappointing in that the central nervous system proved unable to deal with such disruption but there proved to be an unexpected finding. The muscles used were the soleus and the extensor digitorum longus of the cat (respectively, red and white muscles) and at the end of the experiment it was noticed that the re-innervated muscles had changed colour. When tested it was found that they had also changed their contractile characteristics (Fig. 4.7).

This experiment has now been repeated many times and it is clear that the histochemical and contractile properties of muscle fibres are determined by the nerve supplying the muscle. The question then arose as to what feature of the innervation was important. Was some growth factor passing down the nerve from the motoneurone or was the determining factor the activity pattern which the nerve imposed on the muscle?

Salmons & Vrbova (1969) implanted electrodes around the motor nerve serving a fast muscle (extensor digitorum longus) in the rabbit and stimulated at low frequency for several hours a day. After 30 days this fast muscle came to resemble the slow soleus muscle in its appearance and contractile characteristics. The same workers later demonstrated that the presence of the nerve itself is not required since, if conduction along the nerve is blocked and the muscle is stimulated directly, the change from fast to slow characteristics still occurs. These experiments indicate that it is the pattern of activity imposed on the muscle, rather than trophic substances coming from the nerve, that regulates the expression of genes coding for proteins responsible for the slow contractile properties.

The rationale for using prolonged low-frequency stimulation was that this reflects the type of electrical activity that can be recorded from slow muscles which are normally active. In general, slow muscles are used for minor adjustments of posture and position and are consequently required to be continuously active, making frequent small contractions while the animal is awake. In contrast, fast muscles have a pattern of activity where they are electrically silent for long periods and then discharge with short high-frequency bursts as the animal makes occasional rapid or high-force contractions. It now appears, however, that it is not the frequency itself that is of prime importance but rather the total duration of the activity. Long periods of high frequency stimulation are equally effective in changing the gene expression.

The major changes seen after chronic stimulation include an increase in capillary density, proliferation of mitochondria, decrease in sarcoplasmic reticulum and the expression of different troponin and myosin isoenzymes which occur with different time courses (Fig. 4.8).

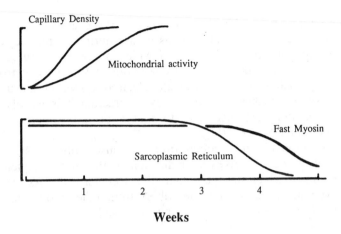

Weeks

Fig. 4.8 Time course of changes with prolonged activity in fast rat or rabbit muscle. Changes in capillary density, mitochondrial content, sarcoplasmic reticulum and alkali stable myosin ATPase as a result of chronic stimulation.

Increased capillary density and mitochondrial content, which are amongst the first changes to be seen in response to prolonged activity, will predominantly affect the fatiguability of the muscle. Changes in the sarcoplasmic reticulum and contractile proteins, which require more activity, influence the speed of the muscle. Although there has been a great deal of work on stimulated animal muscle there are relatively few investigations of the effects of chronic stimulation on human muscle. The studies that have been undertaken show that changes in fatiguability can be produced but that the stimulation has probably never been sufficient to alter the myosin isoenzyme expression, thus converting the type 2 fibres to type 1 (Rutherford & Jones, 1988).

Many top endurance athletes have over 80% type 1 fibres in their leg muscles and there is considerable debate as to whether they were born this way or have achieved the fibre type disproportion as a result of their prolonged training. Human stimulation studies have continued for only a few months, while most endurance athletes, by the time they reach the highest levels, have been training intensively for many years. On the other hand, studies of identical twins have shown that there is a

strong genetic influence over fibre type proportions as there is for
maximum aerobic exercise capacity (VO_2Max) which is determined, in
part, by the fibre type composition (see Chapter 7, Section 7.3.3).

4.5 Motor unit recruitment

Motor units vary in their size and contractile characteristics and these
differences reflect different patterns of use during normal activity.

Information about the order in which motor units are recruited in
human muscle can be obtained by recording EMG activity from single
motor units using fine wire or needle electrodes inserted into the muscle.
As the subject makes a small steady contraction it is usually possible,
by manipulating the electrode, to find a position where a dominant
persistent spike is seen (Fig. 4.9).

The dominant spike comes from the muscle fibre closest to the tip
of the electrode and gives an indication of the firing frequency of the
motor unit of which that particular fibre forms a part. As the electrode
is moved about in the muscle, fibres from other motor units can be
identified and their pattern of firing examined.

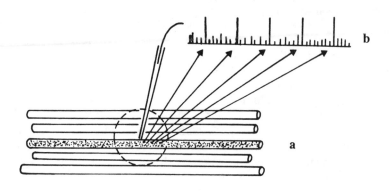

Fig. 4.9 Recording single motor unit activity. **a**, needle electrode with tip close to
one fibre. **b**, electrical activity recorded from a number of fibres but with one fibre
(shaded) giving a large regular spike.

Motor units become active at characteristic levels of force. As the
force increases unit A (Fig. 4.10) is recruited at a low threshold and

fires at a low frequency; unit B is recruited at a greater force and fires at a higher frequency.

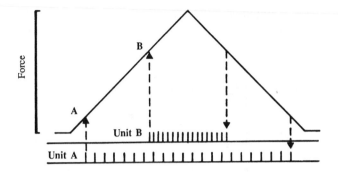

Fig. 4.10 Recruitment of two motor units at different forces. The upper line is the record of force and the lower two lines the activity recorded by two separate microelectrodes. Unit A has a low force threshold, while Unit B is recruited at a higher force.

The force contribution of a single unit will be superimposed on force generated by other active units which are firing more or less randomly. If the EMG signal from a single unit can be identified it can be used to trigger a signal averager so that the contribution of force from the one unit can be identified, and its size and contractile characteristics measured. The low threshold units prove to be small, slow, motor units, while those recruited at higher thresholds are larger fast units (Yemm, 1977).

There appears to be an ordered recruitment of motor units, with small slow motor units being recruited during low-force contractions while the fast units are active only during high-force contractions. Henneman and co workers found that in the cat small, slow motor units were supplied by small, easily excitable motoneurones, while larger units were innervated by motoneurones that had higher thresholds for excitation. Henneman suggested that this difference might be the basis for the modulation of force, with units being recruited in order of size. This has become known as *Henneman's size principle* (Henneman *et al*, 1974). By progressive recruitment of motor units the force generated in a muscle can be increased in a stepwise fashion. At low forces the steps are small (small motor units) giving a smooth increase in force while at higher forces the increments are larger, since the recruited motor units are larger, and consequently control is less precise (Fig. 4.11).

The recruitment pattern described above has advantages in that the most frequently used units are small, slow and fatigue resistant and can provide fine control for the majority of everyday activities such as postural adjustments which require relatively small forces. The large fast and rapidly fatiguable units are only used for occasional high force contractions such as sprinting or jumping where fine control is not necessary.

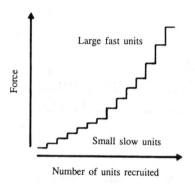

Fig. 4.11 Regulation of force by recruitment. Small motor units are recruited first with the larger units coming in at the higher forces.

An alternative way of modulating force is to vary the frequency of stimulation (see Fig. 4.3); this is known as rate coding. It is not known to what extent these two methods of varying force, recruitment and rate coding are used during a normal voluntary contraction. It is possible that in a large muscle such as the quadriceps, where fine control is not generally required, force is adjusted by recruitment of motor units which, once recruited, continue firing at a fixed rate. In small muscles like those of the hand where fine control is essential, rate coding may be more important.

4.6 Sensory receptors in skeletal muscle

There are a variety of sensory receptors in muscle. Some of these are nociceptors which signal chemical changes in the muscle (see Chapter 10, Section 10.1), others are concerned with the regulation of force production and muscle length.

4.6.1 *Golgi tendon organs*

Tendon organs are formed by encapsulated endings of large myelinated axons (Ib afferent fibres) situated at musculo-tendinous junctions and are concerned with providing information about muscle tension to the central nervous system. The information from Golgi tendon organs acts via an inhibitory interneurone to reduce the excitability of α- and γ-motoneurones (see Fig. 4.15b). In the cat soleus there are about 50 Golgi tendon organs, and each tendon organ is responsive to a group of muscle fibres closely connected with that portion of tendon. Contraction of only one or two of these fibres can make the tendon organ discharge. Because the fibres of individual motor units are scattered in the muscle, it may be any one of a number of motor units which drives the tendon organ at any one time.

4.6.2 *Muscle spindles*

Spindles are found scattered throughout a muscle, some in the belly and others near the musculo-tendinous junctions (Boyd, 1976). Each spindle consists of a number of highly specialised muscle fibres contained within a collagenous capsule; these fibres are described as *intrafusal* fibres as opposed to the vast majority of muscle fibres which are *extrafusal*. A diagrammatic representation of a muscle spindle in longitudinal section is shown in Fig. 4.12. There are two types of intrafusal fibre, the larger fibres are about 25μm in diameter and the smaller fibres are less than 20μm.

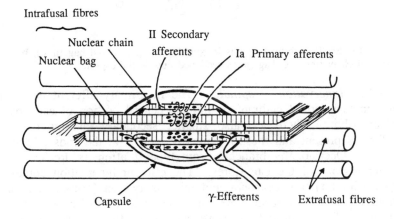

Fig. 4.12 Diagram showing the main features of a muscle spindle. The afferent innervation is only shown for the upper chain and bag fibres while the efferent innervation is shown for the lower fibres.

All the intrafusal fibres are smaller than the extrafusal fibres, being half their diameter or less. The length of a spindle in a cat muscle is about 7-10mm. In the central region of the larger fibres there is a cluster (bag) of 50-100 nuclei; fibres of this type have been designated *bag fibres*. The nuclei of the smaller fibres form a central chain and these fibres have come to be known as *chain fibres*.

A cross-section in the central area of a spindle will show a group of nuclei in bag fibres but only one nucleus in a chain fibre (Fig. 4.13, see also Fig. 1.17). The chain fibres are attached to the bag fibres within the capsule. The bag fibres extend beyond the capsule and are attached to extrafusal fibres, often to different fibres at each end. The capsule is filled with clear lymph.

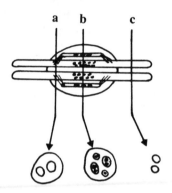

Fig. 4.13 Sections through a muscle spindle. **a**, capsule and bag fibres; **b**, capsule, bag and chain fibres; **c**, bag fibres sectioned outside the capsule.

4.6.2.1 *Innervation of spindles* The Ia primary afferent nerve fibres terminate in spiral endings around the central portion of each bag and chain fibre. There are also smaller secondary endings of type II afferents present and these are mainly located at the ends of the chain fibres. Occasionally branches from type II afferents are seen on the outer regions of the bag fibres. The efferent innervation comes from γ- (fusimotor) motoneurones and this innervation forms synapses with both types of intrafusal fibre on either side of the central nucleated portion. The chain and bag fibres are similar to extrafusal fibres in the arrangement and function of their contractile proteins but they differ in that they do not generate propagated action potentials, contraction being localised to regions on either side of the central nucleated portions. When the γ-motoneurones cause the fibres to contract the effect is therefore to stretch the central portion of the intrafusal fibres around which the primary nerve endings are situated (see Fig. 4.16).

4.6.2.2 *Response to stretch*   In response to a ramp and hold stretch there is a rapid increase in the frequency of firing in the primary Ia afferents originating on the bag fibres (Fig. 4.14).   During the hold phase when the spindle is at a constant length the rate of firing decreases. Bag fibres are said to *accommodate* to the stretch and therefore act mainly as indicators of *rate of change*.

The chain fibres behave in a more *elastic fashion* and give a sustained high frequency response during the hold phase.   This signal is mainly from the secondary endings (type II afferents) but there are also primary afferents on the chain fibres so that the signal in the type Ia afferents may be a mixture derived from the responses from both types of intrafusal fibre.

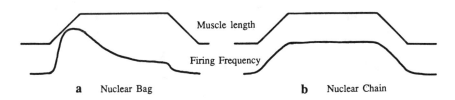

a   Nuclear Bag   b   Nuclear Chain

Fig. 4.14 The response of intrafusal fibres to stretch. **a**, the bag fibres accommodate to stretch, while, **b**, the chain fibres remain stretched and continue to fire.

4.6.2.3 *Input to the central nervous system* The primary and secondary afferents have their cell bodies in the dorsal root ganglia and have excitatory synaptic inputs to the α-motoneurones supplying the muscle in which the spindles are situated.

Spindles function as stretch receptors in a servo loop controlling length or tension in a muscle.   Stretch of the spindle causes afferent discharge which activates the α-motoneurones causing contraction of the muscle: an example of this is the simple stretch reflex (Fig. 4.15a). Not only do the spindle afferents feed back to the α-motoneurones of the muscle in which they are situated, they also have a synaptic input to the α-motoneurones of antagonist muscles where they exert an inhibitory influence (Fig. 4.15b). This inhibition ensures that antagonist muscles do not work against one another.

Intrafusal fibres are innervated by axonal branches from the γ-motoneurones in the spinal cord (Fig. 4.15b). When the γ-motoneurone fires the two ends of each intrafusal fibre contract stretching the central portion and activating the primary and secondary afferent endings. The afferent activity stimulates the α-motoneurones causing the extrafusal fibres to contract: when these fibres shorten the stretch on the intrafusal fibres is removed and the afferent signal is reduced (Fig. 4.16).

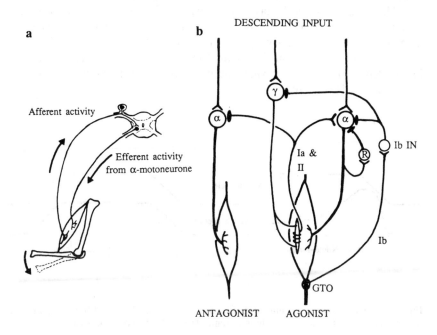

Fig. 4.15 Spinal stretch reflex. **a**, simple reflex; afferent activity activates the α-motoneurone causing contraction of the extrafusal muscle fibres. **b**, more complex wiring diagram of the α- and γ-innervation and the afferent inputs modifying their activity. Y-shaped endings indicate excitatory synapses, solid endings, inhibitory synapses.   GTO, Golgi tendon organ; R, Renshaw cell; Ib IN, Ib inhibitory interneurone.

The system therefore acts to maintain a muscle at a given length; if the whole muscle is stretched the muscle spindle afferent input to the motoneurones will cause the muscle to contract back to its original length. Alternatively activity in the γ-motoneurones can be used to set the muscle length, the higher the activity the shorter the length.

The extent to which normal movements are controlled by the activity of α- or γ-motoneurones is not known. There have been suggestions that small low force postural movements may involve activation of the γ-motoneurones whereas rapid movements are the result of direct descending activation of α-motoneurones. Alternatively, or in other situations, there may be co-activation of α- and γ-motoneurones. Activity of the γ-motoneurones will make the spindles more responsive to stretch and increase the sensitivity of the servo loop thereby giving greater control during a movement.

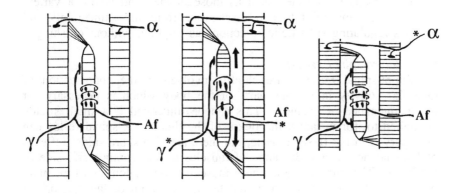

Fig. 4.16 Action of muscle spindles. **a**, starting position; **b**, γ-activity (*) stretches the central portion of the spindle (arrows) causing afferent discharge (*), **c**, α-motoneurone activity (*) causes contraction of extrafusal fibres, shortening of spindle and reduced afferent discharge. **Af**, afferent fibres (type Ia or II).

The Ia and II afferent inputs from the spindles are important in controlling motoneurone activity exerting a strong excitatory influence, but there are many other modulating influences, including Renshaw cell (small interneurones in the spinal cord that receive colateral input) inhibition and descending pathways affecting the excitability of the α-motoneurones via inhibitory interneurones (Fig. 4.15b). The Ib Golgi tendon organ afferent activity exerts an inhibitory effect on α- and γ-motoneurones. Information also comes to the central nervous system from pressure receptors in the skin and nociceptors in the muscle and fascial sheath which respond to metabolite changes in the active muscle and may exert an inhibitory influence on α-motoneurones (Fournier & Pierrot-Deseilligny, 1989).

4.7 Reflex activity

Reflex activity may either traverse a relatively short spinal pathway or take a longer path via the higher centres in the brain. These two kinds of reflex can be identified by their latency, that is, the time taken for a signal to traverse the reflex arc. For spinal reflexes this time is of the order of 10-20msec, while for supra-spinal reflexes it is 50msec or more (Marsden *et al*, 1976).

4.7.1 *Spinal reflexes*
Spinal reflexes play an important role in coordinating the activity of local groups of muscles such as those in the hand where a variety of excitatory and inhibitory reflexes arise from the skin, joints and muscles regulating such delicate actions as gripping without crushing.

4.7.2 *Supra-spinal reflexes*
Supra-spinal reflexes are chiefly involved in the coordination of muscular activity in various parts of the body which is necessary for the maintenance of balance. This can be illustrated if a small stretch is applied to, for instance, the flexor of the thumb. A spinal reflex can be observed in the flexor muscle, but there are also supra-spinal reflexes of long latency in a wide range of muscles on the contralateral side of the body. The importance of these muscular contractions is to maintain balance so that the subject does not fall as the result of the pull on his thumb. Without these compensating contractions even the simplest movement of lifting a cup would unbalance the body. Since man has a highly unstable form of locomotion, the maintenance of posture and balance constitutes a most important role for these reflexes.

4.8 Coordination of muscular contractions

All bodily movements, while usually seeming quite simple for a healthy adult, nevertheless involve highly complex patterns of muscular contraction.   These movements are generally made without any consciousness of the complexity or even the contraction sequence of the various muscles used. For a task such as reaching out to pick up a cup the simplest sequence of muscle commands must include:
1.   Activate elbow extensors - arm extends
2.   Activate finger extensors - hand opens
3.   Activate finger flexors - cup is grasped
4.   Activate elbow flexors - cup is brought up towards body.
For a very young child this would represent a major achievement requiring great concentration to activate the right muscles in the correct sequence. With time and practice the conscious command "pick up that

cup" serves to initiate the correct sequence of movements without conscious effort. This problem may be thought of in terms of robotics or computer control in which the sequence 1-4 above would be stored as a subroutine to be called up whenever the appropriate movement is required. Nearly every action in the daily life of an adult is encoded in this way and it is only when we encounter an unfamiliar activity such as writing with our non-dominant hand, or learning to ski or to ride a bicycle as an adult that we become conscious of the complex learning process involved. We also see again the grim determination and concentration that is required to learn the new task.

It is of particular interest to know where in the central nervous system these subroutines are located. In insects, various locomotor and other functions have been localised to specific neuronal groups. In higher animals locomotor activity is integrated with other bodily activities and it is not easy to identify discrete locomotor centres (Armstrong, 1988). There are, however, some situations where activities or movements can be demonstrated to be under the control of the spinal cord and independent of the higher motor centres. A decapitated chicken will continue to run about for some time and complex locomotor movements can be demonstrated in decerebrate cats and dogs if the body is supported over a moving treadmill. These preparations will also show a scratch reflex in response to stimulation of the skin in the lumbar region. Locomotion in cats and dogs is a complex task involving the co-ordination of many muscle groups in 4 separate limbs. Moreover the pattern of locomotion will change in response to changes in treadmill speed. The computing power to achieve this must be considerable and must exist within the spinal cord.

A parallel situation in man is seen when the spinal cord has become separated from the higher motor centres by some injury. Such paraplegic patients, however, do not show automatic locomotor reflexes. This observation indicates that human locomotion requires some input from the higher centres, although this input need not necessarily be conscious. It may also reflect the fact that an upright posture is much more demanding in terms of co-ordination than four-legged locomotion, and balancing an unstable body on two legs requires the greater computing power available in the higher motor centres just as modern high performance aircraft are inherently unstable and require sophisticated computer control to keep them flying.

It may still, however, be over-simplistic to think of the movement subroutines in terms of specific instructions concerning individual muscles. This is suggested by an observation described by P.A. Merton (1972). He noticed that when he wrote his signature in very small letters using a magnifying glass and a mapping pen it was recognizably the same as when he wrote it large on a wall. The specific muscles used to perform these two tasks were very different, in the first case small delicate movements by the hand muscles and in the second large bold movements of the whole arm and shoulder. Despite this, the signature was characteristically his own in both cases suggesting that the final control is situated in some higher central area and exists in a very much more complex form than a mere sequence of muscle movements.

4.9　References and further reading

Armstrong, D.M. (1988). The supraspinal control of mammalian locomotion. *Journal of Physiology* **405**, 1-38.

Boyd, I.A. (1976). The mechanical properties of dynamic nuclear bag fibres, static nuclear bag fibres and nuclear chain fibres in isolated cat muscle spindles. *Progress in Brain Research* **44**, 33-50.

Buller, A.J., Eccles, J.C. & Eccles, R.M. (1960). Interactions between motor neurnones and muscles in respect of the characteristic speeds of their responses. *Journal of Physiology* **150**, 417-39.

Burke, R.E., Levine, D.M., Tsairis, P. & Aajai, F.E. (1973). Physiological types and histological profiles in motor units of cat gastrocnemius. *Journal of Physiology* **234**, 723-48.

Burke, R.E., Levine, D.M., Zajac, F.E., Tsairis, P. & Engel, W.K. (1971). Mammalian motor units: physiological-histochemical correlation in three types in cat gastrocnemius. *Science* **174**, 709-12.

Dubowitz, V. (1985). *Muscle Biopsy, a Practical Approach,* 2nd edition. London, Baillière Tindall.

Fournier, E. & Pierrot-Deseilligny, E. (1989). Changes in transmission in some reflex pathways during movement in humans. *News in Physiological Sciences* **4**, 29-32.

Garnett, R.A.F., O'Donovan, M.J., Stephens, J.A. & Taylor, A. (1979). Motor unit organization of human medial gastrocnemius. *Journal of Physiology* **287**, 33-43.

Henneman, E., Clamann, H.P., Gillies, J.D. & Skinner, R.D. (1974). Rank order of motoneurons within a pool, law of combination. *Journal of Neurophysiology* **37**, 1338-49.

Kugelberg, E. (1973). Histochemical composition, contraction speed and fatiguability of rat soleus motor units. *Journal of the Neurological Sciences* **20**, 177-98.

Marsden, C.D., Merton, P.A. & Morton, H.B. (1976). Stretch reflex and servo action in a variety of human muscles. *Journal of Physiology* **259**, 531-60.

Marsden, C.D., Merton, P.A. & Morton, H.B. (1977). The sensory mechanism of servo action in human muscle. *Journal of Physiology* **265**, 521-35.

Merton, P.A. (1972). How we control the contraction of our muscles. *Scientific American* **226**, 30-7.

Peter, J.B., Barnard, V.R., Edgerton, V.R., Gillespie, C.A. & Stempel, K.E. (1972). Metabolic profiles of three fibre types of skeletal muscles in guinea pigs and rabbits. *Biochemistry* **11**, 2627-33.

Ranvier, M.L. (1873). Propriétés et structures différentes des muscles rouges et des muscles blancs, chez les Lapins et chez les Raies. *Comptes Rendus des Académie de Sciences* **77**, 1030-4.

Rutherford, O.M. & Jones, D.A. (1988). Contractile properties and fatiguability of the human adductor pollicis and first dorsal interosseus: a comparison of the effects of two chronic stimulation patterns. *Journal of the Neurological Sciences* **85**, 319-31.

Salmons, S. & Henriksson, K. (1981). The adaptive response of skeletal muscle to increased use. *Muscle & Nerve* **4**, 94-105.

Salmons, S. & Vrbova, G. (1969). The influence of activity on some contractile characteristics of mammalian fast and slow muscles. *Journal of Physiology* **201**, 535-49.

Yemm, R. (1977). The orderly recruitment of motor units of the masseter and temporal muscles during voluntary isometric contractions in man. *Journal of Physiology* **265**, 163-74.

Chapter 5

GROWTH, DEVELOPMENT AND AGEING OF MUSCLE

From the infant, through childhood, adolesence, adulthood and old age, there are considerable changes in the extent and patterns of physical activity which are reflected in changes in the quality and quantity of skeletal muscle.

5.1 Embryonic origins and foetal development

Skeletal muscle is derived from the embryonic mesoderm. In about the sixth week of gestation there is a condensation of the mesenchyme and mesodermal stem cells begin to differentiate to form myoblasts. Some myoblasts remain as single cells with mitotic potential and these will form the satellite cells. Other myoblasts aggregate and fuse to form primary myotubes attached at each end to the tendons and the developing skeleton. Within the developing myotube a central chain of nuclei forms (Fig. 5.1), surrounded by basophilic cytoplasm rich in polyribosomes.

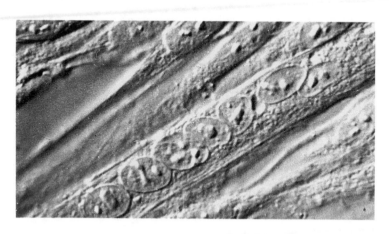

Fig. 5.1 Cultured myoblasts fuse to form myotubes: note the chain of central nuclei.

Mid-way along the primary myotubes further myoblasts aggregate and fuse to form secondary myotubes. At first the primary and secondary myotubes share a common basement membrane (Fig. 5.2a) but eventually the secondary myotubes develop a separate basement membrane, make contact with the tendon and become independent of the primaries. In the human foetus the transition from myoblasts to primary myotube takes place in around the seventh to ninth weeks of gestation and by the end of this period the primordia of most muscle groups are well defined. At this time the synthesis of the contractile proteins, actin and myosin, begins and the first signs of cross striation are visible (Fig. 5.2b).

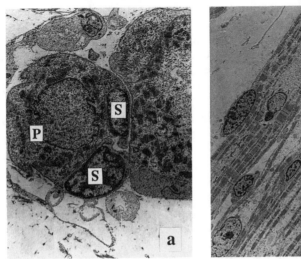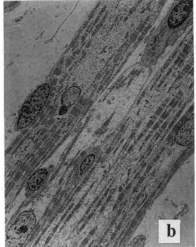

Fig. 5.2 Developing myotubes and fibres. **a**, primary myotube (**P**) with two attached myoblasts forming the secondary myotubes (**S**); note that they are contained within the same basement membrane; 12 weeks gestation. **b**, longitudinal section of myotubes showing the formation of myofibrils; 12 weeks gestation.

From 11 weeks onwards there is a proliferation of myofibrils leading to hypertrophy of the muscle fibres which also grow in length by the addition of sarcomeres at the ends. At 16 to 17 weeks a further population of myotubes becomes apparent and are known as the tertiary myotubes. These myotubes are small, adhere close to the secondary myotubes and are enclosed within the same basement membrane. By 18 to 23 weeks the tertiary myotubes have become independent and the nuclei of the more mature myotubes begin to move to the periphery of the fibre. Under the light microscope it is very difficult to distinguish muscle fibre nuclei from the 5% to 10% of nuclei that belong to satellite cells. With the electron microscope the position of the satellite cells beneath the basement membrane, but outside the plasma membrane, of the muscle can be seen (see Fig.1.16). If the muscle fibre is damaged the satellite cells are activated to divide and begin the process of regeneration.

The developing fibres express a number of different myosins which can be identified with monoclonal antibodies: these include an embryonic form and an intermediate fast type that confers the properties of the type 2c fibres (often seen in regenerating adult muscle) when stained for myosin ATPase. The primary myotubes can be identified throughout embryonic development as they alone express adult slow myosin from about 9 weeks of gestation (Drager *et al*, 1987). At around 10 weeks the nervous system makes contact with the developing muscle fibres and, in response to the contractile activity imposed by the motor nerve, the fibres slowly differentiate so that, eventually, foetal myosins are no longer expressed and about 50% of fibres express slow myosin and 50% fast myosin (see Chapters 3 & 4). This process, which is apparent by about 32 weeks of gestation, is probably not fully completed in human muscle until a few months after birth.

5.2 Size of adult muscle

The number of fibres in each human muscle is probably set by 24 weeks of gestation. In the rat, fibre numbers do not change during life while the mean fibre cross-sectional area increases nearly tenfold from the newborn to adult animal (Rowe & Goldspink, 1969). There are considerable practical and ethical problems involved in making measurements of fibre size and number in children and adults but the limited data available suggest that there is an increase in size without a change in fibre numbers (hypertrophy without hyperplasia) as the muscles grow in size and strength. Adult muscle fibre cross-sectional areas are reached shortly after puberty (Fig. 5.3). In an adult man about 40-45% of the body weight is muscle and this figure is slightly lower in females. The mean cross-sectional area of fibres in a biopsy from the quadriceps muscle in a normal man is about 3,500-7,500 μm^2 and in normal women from 2,000 to 5,000 μm^2.

Skeletal muscle contains a large proportion of the body creatine, a small fraction of which spontaneously forms the anhydride, creatinine, with the two ends of the creatine molecule forming a peptide link (Fig. 5.4). Creatinine, which has no biological function, passes into the plasma where it is filtered by the kidney and not reabsorbed; creatinine clearance being the classic test of glomerular filtration rate.

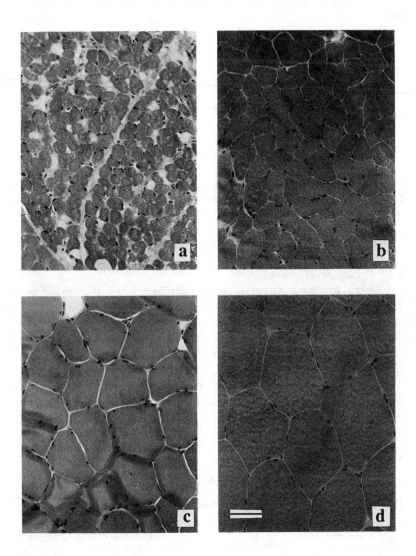

Fig. 5.3 Growth of muscle fibre size of the human quadriceps. **a**, baby aged 8 months. **b**, child of 5 years. **c**, boy, aged 14. **d**, large male, aged 23. All at the same magnification and stained with haematoxylin & eosin. Bar in **d** = 50μm.

The amount of creatinine produced in a day is related to the total body content of creatine (mainly muscle) and the 24 hour excretion in the urine is, therefore, an indicator of muscle mass. Fifty to seventy per cent of body potassium is contained in muscle so that measurement of whole body potassium is also a useful way of estimating lean body mass.

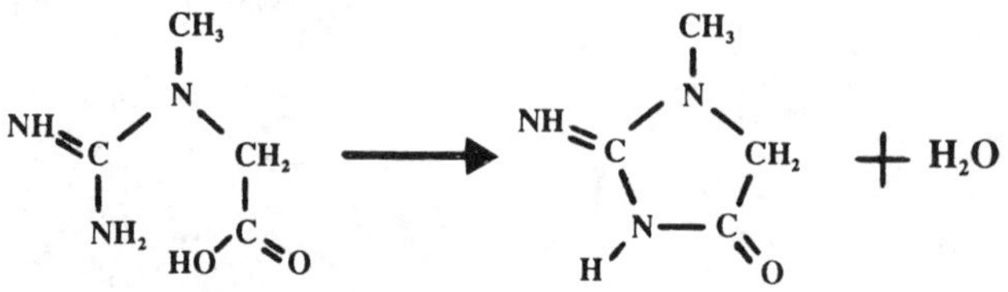

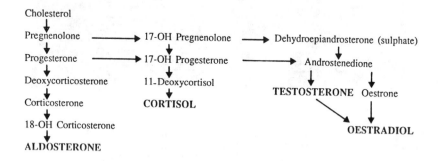

Fig. 5.4 The formation of creatinine from muscle creatine.

5.3 Endocrine influences on growth and development

5.3.1 *Foetal development*

Current evidence suggests that most hormones that regulate cell division and maturation in the adult, including *growth hormone*, thyroid hormones, *insulin* and *prolactin* do not cross the placenta in physiologically important amounts. Cortisol does pass but is largely converted into inactive cortisone by the placenta. The direct hormonal influences on the developing foetus are, therefore, placental and foetal in origin. The placenta and the foetal adrenal glands act as a co-ordinated endocrine organ during foetal life forming what is sometimes termed the *foetoplacental* unit.

Cholesterol
↓
Pregnenolone ⟶ 17-OH Pregnenolone ⟶ Dehydroepiandrosterone (sulphate)
↓   ↓
Progesterone ⟶ 17-OH Progesterone ⟶ Androstenedione
↓   ↓   ↓   ↓
Deoxycorticosterone   11-Deoxycortisol   **TESTOSTERONE** Oestrone
↓   ↓
Corticosterone   **CORTISOL**
↓   ↓
18-OH Corticosterone   **OESTRADIOL**
↓
ALDOSTERONE

Fig. 5.5 The metabolism of steroid hormones.

The placenta produces pregnenolone which is processed by the foetal adrenal cortex to produce androgens (mainly dehydro-epiandrosterone sulphate) which return to the placenta and are processed to form oestrogens (see Fig. 5.5). Most of the oestrogen formed passes back into the maternal circulation and acts to maintain the pregnancy, supressing ovarian function and ensuring the placental blood supply and good foetal nutrition. Towards term the adrenal production of androgens falls as the production of corticosteroids rises.

The anterior lobe of the foetal pituitary secretes a *thyrotrophic hormone* that stimulates the thyroid gland to produce *thyroxine*. Thyroxine is important in growth and maturation, particularly of the brain, and establishing the connection between muscle and nerve.

Growth hormone is another product of the anterior lobe of the pituitary. This polypeptide hormone can be detected in the foetus by the eighth to tenth week of gestation soon after the pituitary has been formed. Although growth hormone appears early in gestation it does not seem to be essential for foetal growth; it is mainly after birth that children lacking growth hormone fail to grow normally. The role of pituitary growth hormone is largely fulfilled in foetal life by one of the major hormones produced by the placenta, *human placental lactogen* (hPL). As with growth hormone, hPL, although having some direct activity, acts mainly via the paracrine *insulin-like growth factors* 1 and 2 (IGF1, IGF2). Peptide growth factors, which include *platelet-derived growth factor, epithelial growth factor, IGF1* and *IGF2*, are closely associated with early embryological differentiation and subsequent foetal growth. It is possible that the IGFs are present and biologically active from the pre-implantation stage; they are synthesised by a variety of foetal cell types, particularly human foetal myoblasts, hepatocytes and chondrocytes. Although they may be produced as a result of stimulation by hPL there is also evidence for spontaneous production by all the above tissues.

The maximum rate of growth in height (length) of the foetus occurs at about 16 weeks of gestation but at birth the rate of growth is still faster than at any other time during postnatal life.

5.3.2 *Sexual development of the foetus*

Sex is determined by the sex chomosome combination in the fertilized ovum, XX being female and XY male. The sex of an individual has a considerable influence on their physical development. Male babies are born, on average, 150g heavier than girls and, as adults, men are generally larger than women with a greater proportion of skeletal muscle. In addition, the more aggressive behaviour patterns that frequently accompany the Y chromosome tend to accentuate the differences in size when it comes to physical activity and contact sports.

Genes on the short arm of the Y chromosome code for the histocompatability -Y antigen (H-Y), a surface antigen which forces the primordial gonad to develop into a testis. Without the H-Y antigen the natural development is to express the female phenotype. *Human chorionic gonadotrophin* (hCG), secreted by the placenta, has a similar action to that of gonadotrophin in the adult and, in the male foetus, stimulates the Leydig cells of the testis to produce testosterone. The foetal testis also produces *anti-mullerian hormone* which, together with testoserone, causes the regression of the Mullerian duct, the development of the Wollfian duct and of the external male genitalia. In the absence of anti-mullerian hormone, Mullerian ducts persist and the female genital tract is formed. In contrast to the male gonad the foetal ovary seems to be largely inactive and plays little or no part in foetal development.

5.3.3 *Postnatal development*

After birth there is a surge of *leutenising hormone* (LH) in both sexes which persists for several months and in male infants there is a marked rise in plasma testosterone with values approaching adult levels. In rats this surge of testosterone in important in determining the subsequent pattern of growth and sexual behaviour. It is possible that the high testosterone level in human male babies has a similar function, predisposing the male to certain growth and behaviour patterns. Within one year of birth, however, the hypothalamic pituitary axis becomes quiescent probably as a result of neural influences in which the pineal may be involved.

The hypothalamus and anterior pituitary glands play a key role in controlling growth (Fig. 5.6). All the anterior pituitary hormones are secreted in a pulsatile fashion in response to the intermittent release of the appropriate releasing hormone from the hypothalamus. Growth hormone (GH) is under the control of *growth hormone-releasing hormone* (GHRH) and the *gonadotrophins, leutenising hormone* (LH) and *follicle stimulating hormone* (FSH) are controlled by *gonadotrophin-releasing hormone* (GnRH). The pulsatile nature of the secretion appears to be most important for hormone action and in conditions where hormone replacement therapy is required, divided doses provide the most efficient form of replacement, indeed gonadotrophin-releasing hormone, used to induce puberty, is ineffective when given as a steady infusion.

Growth hormone release increases in a variety of circumstances including raised circulating levels of oestradiol, sleep, exercise and the ingestion of high concentrations of basic amino acids such as ornithine and arginine. This unusual combination of factors probably reflects the fact that GH has at least two functions, one as a promotor of growth, the other is as a hormone regulating the use of fat and carbohydrate during exercise.

In its growth-promoting function, GH acts through intermediary paracrine hormones, mainly somatomedins, or insulin-like growth factors,

IGF1 and IGF2. IGF2 is important in embryonic growth and development but its postnatal role is uncertain. IGF1 is produced in the target tissues; in muscle the GH receptors may be on the muscle fibre and/or on associated fibroblasts. The latter have been shown to secrete IGF1 in response to growth hormone *in vitro*. The production of IGF1 is inhibited by poor nutrition. IGF1 and insulin are very similar proteins and both have an important role in maintaining protein synthesis in muscle. The name "insulin-like growth factor" reflects this similarity in structure and function.

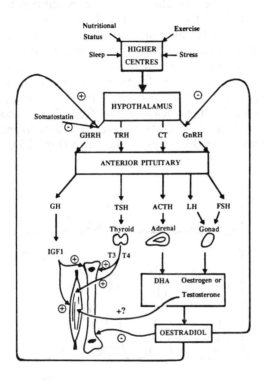

Fig. 5.6 Hormones of the hypothalamus and anterior pituitary and their action in respect to growth of muscle and bone. Oestradiol has a negative feedback on GnRH production but stimulates GHRH release. The direct action of testosterone on muscle is speculative.

Corticosteroids suppress the production of growth hormone and IGF1 and it is well known that young patients receiving corticosteroid therapy fail to grow at a normal rate. Restoration of growth occurs if the steroids are discontinued.

5.3.3 *Endocrine changes during puberty*

During puberty there is a rapid increase in body size and a commensurate increase in muscle bulk as a result of the complex endocrine changes that take place at this time.

The initial endocrine event of puberty appears to be an increase in the nocturnal secretion of LH from the pituitary in response to pulsatile secretion of GnRH from the hypothalamus. In the young child there are occasional bursts of GnRH but regular secretion does not occur until the start of puberty. During the early stages of puberty secretion occurs at night, largely in association with REM sleep, while in the later stages high amplitude pulsatile secretion also occurs during the day. LH stimulates the growth of the gonads and the production of testosterone by the Leydig cells in boys and, in girls, the production of oestrogen by the aromatisation of androstendione. Consequently the circulating levels of testosterone or oestrogen are increased. Oestrogen and testosterone are responsible for the development of the secondary sexual characteristics and also, after conversion to oestradiol, potentiate the action of GHRH so that the release of GH from the anterior pituitary is increased. The frequency of the GH pulses increases to reach a peak at around puberty and then decreases in the adult (Fig. 5.7).

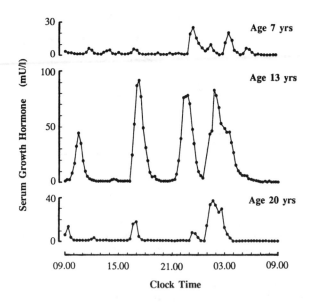

Fig. 5.7 24 hour profile of growth hormone release in males of different ages (courtesy of Dr P. Hindmarsh).

It is GH, probably acting through IGF1, and TSH acting via the thyroid hormones, that stimulate muscle and bone growth. The pubertal growth spurt in girls occurs at an earlier stage of sexual development because oestrogen is a more potent inducer of GHRH production by the hypothalamus, with the consequent increase in GH release, than is testosterone which must be converted to oestradiol before becoming active in this respect (Link *et al*, 1986). It is of interest that circulating levels of insulin also increase during puberty, possibly to facilitate transport of amino acids to support rapid tissue growth. By 14 or 15 years of age most girls have achieved their adult height while in boys, final height is not reached until about 16 or 17 years. Growth of the long bones ceases with closure of the epiphyseal growth plates as a consequence of the high circulating levels of sex steroids.

The mechanisms that determine the timing of puberty are of considerable interest but are poorly understood. The increased pulsatile secretion of GnRH is the primary cause of the onset of puberty but there is dispute as to the reason for the change in hypothalamic function that gives rise to the increased production.

From the age of 8 or 9 the adrenal cortex secretes increasing quantities of androgens (adrenache), with adult levels of adrenal androgen secretion being reached in the early stages of puberty. The main adrenal androgen is dihydoepiandrosterone (DHA), a small portion of which is converted to testosterone and oestradiol. There have been suggestions that increasing adrenal androgens cause the hypothalamus to "mature" and begin the pulsatile secretion of GnRH; however, this now seems unlikely. Adrenal androgens may be involved in the growth of pubic and axial hair in girls, but oestrogens seem to be required for full development.

It has become evident that the increase in pulsatile GnRH secretion is an event controlled by some inherent timing set by the central nervous system and that it is not triggered by other hormonal changes. Thus in young rhesus monkeys, puberty can be induced by giving GnRH in a pulsatile fashion but, on withdrawl of treatment, the monkeys revert to a pre-pubertal state only to have a natural puberty at the appropriate time. Experience of children with delayed puberty treated with pulsatile GnRH suggests that a similar mechanism may operate during human adolescence. The timing of pulstile GnRH release is under the control of a group of neurones in the arcuate nucleus of the hypothalamus but it is not known what perturbs this timing to initiate the start of puberty. It is possible that the pineal gland may be active in this respect as pineal tumours may be associated with disturbances of pubertal onset.

5.3.4 *Endocrine changes with ageing*

Testosterone, whether derived from the testes or from adrenal androgens, can be aromatised to oestradiol at a variety of sites including adipose tissue, but this is not a major pathway and males have consistently lower levels of oestradiol than females. In women after the menopause, ovarian oestradiol disappears and the only remaining source is that produced from adrenal androgens. Older women, therefore, have lower oestradiol levels than men who continue to have available both testicular and adrenal testosterone to convert into oestradiol. Consequently, whilst young women tend to have higher peaks of growth hormone than young men, the situation is reversed in older men and women. It is notable that after the menopause women show considerable muscle wasting and become much more susceptible to osteoporosis than do men. The post-menopausal thinning of bone which leads to osteoporosis can be minimised by oestrogen replacement therapy (although it is not yet known whether the muscle also responds) and this suggests a continuing role for the sex steroids, and probably growth hormone, in maintaining bone and muscle bulk throughout life.

5.4 Strength and muscle mass

The development of muscle is usually assessed by increases in voluntary strength. The difficulty with this measurement is that it is important to separate increases in muscle size from improvements in skill and co-ordination which all lead to an increase in performance.

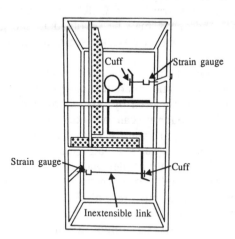

Fig. 5.8 Simple apparatus for measuring isometric strength of the quadriceps and elbow flexors. The subject is firmly held in the chair with a strap around the hips.

To assess muscular strength by itself it is necessary to have tests that require only the minimum of skill (Fig. 5.8) and, even so, it is difficult to make accurate measurements of strength in young children. However, after the age of 5 or 6 reliable measurements can be made and there is a steady and similar increase in strength in both sexes up to the age of puberty when, during the growth spurt and sexual maturation, a more rapid increase occurs (Fig. 5.9).

In the years before puberty, muscles of the lower limbs grow in proportion to the body weight (or height cubed). Teliologically this might be expected as muscles in the leg clearly have the function of bearing the body weight. Muscles in the upper body, however, grow less rapidly, in proportion to height squared, the muscles maintaining the same proportions as the long bones increase in length. During puberty and the adolescent growth spurt, the skeletal muscles grow more rapidly in relation to height and body weight (Fig. 5.9).

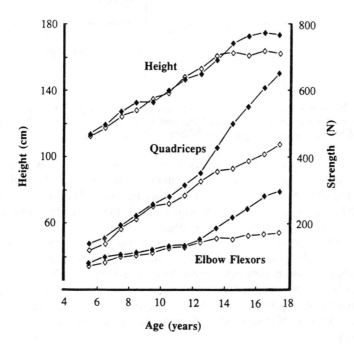

Fig. 5.9 Changes in height and muscle strength with age. Note the steady increase before puberty and, for boys, a rapid increase during, and for a while after, the spurt in height. Open symbols, girls; filled symbols, boys.

For adolescent girls and adult women the proportions of muscle strength to body weight and height remain much the same as those for younger children. In adolescent boys, however, there appears to be an additional stimulus for muscle growth that is particularly noticeable in the muscles of the upper limb girdle. The relationship between strength of the biceps and height differs from that seen in young boys (Fig. 5.10). This additional muscle growth probably represents the direct action of testosterone on muscle.

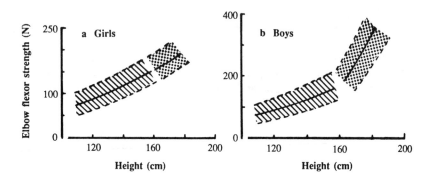

Fig. 5.10 Elbow flexor strength as a function of height. **a**, girls; **b**, boys. The range of values for the shorter prepubertal children is shown cross-hatched. The range for the taller pubertal and postpubertal children is shown dotted.

Most men can manage at least one press-up or chin-up whilst these exercises are very difficult for the majority of women. Throwing, pole vaulting and gymnastic exercises involving strength of the upper body are other activities where men tend to have the advantage over women. It is not clear, however, what evolutionary advantage is gained by one sex having particularly strong arms. The most likely explanation is that it is of little practical advantage but that the upper body muscle development is another male secondary sexual characteristic. The heavy musculature may originally have served the function of either attracting females or of impressing and dominating other males, the latter being the more likely explanation considering the behaviour of other primate species.

5.5 Body proportions (somatotypes)

In addition to differences of height in the adult population it is a matter of common observation that individuals differ in their body proportions (Fig. 5.11). Three basic body types or *somatotypes* have been identified, these are 1, the *ectomorph*, who is "spindly", being thin, with little body fat or muscle, a thin face and long neck. 2, the *mesomorph,* is the chunky, "triangular man" with a large head, broad shoulders and heavily muscled limbs with minimal subcutaneous fat. 3, the *endomorph,* is "pear-shaped" with a round head and a large rounded abdomen predominating over the thorax. There is a great deal of subcutaneous fat, over the upper arm and thigh although the endomorph is not simply fat for if he loses weight he still retains the same overall body proportions.

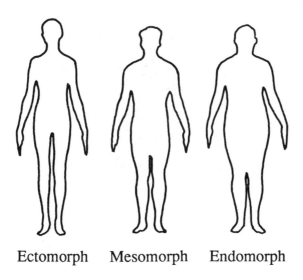

Ectomorph   Mesomorph   Endomorph

Fig. 5.11 The three archetypal male body shapes or somatotypes.

Everybody expresses some elements of each somatotype in their body form, the majority of the population being approximately equal mixtures of all three types.

Interest in somatotypes centres on the fact that there are correlations between somatotype, lifestyle, propensity to disease and sporting ability. Among the male undergraduates at Oxford University in 1948-50 all somatotypes were equally represented while for Physical Education students at Loughborough Training College, there was a complete absence of true endomorphs (Tanner, 1964). Endomorphy appears to be incompatible with (athletic) sporting prowess. Amongst elite athletes certain somatotypes dominate specific events (Fig. 5.12).

One hundred and 200m sprinters are heavily muscled mesomorphs, who, whilst they might be expected to have muscular thighs, also have muscular shoulders and arms. As the track distances increase so the degree of ectomorphy also increases. In jumping events, especially the high jump, most of the competitors are very high in ectomorphy. For the throwing events the competitors are mainly mesomorphic endomorphs with very low ectomorphy scores and are similar in build to the weight lifters. Wrestlers are similar to sprinters and Tanner (1964) comments that the only way of distinguishing the two is by the state of their ears! The differing proportions of muscle to body weight and the lengths of various parts of the skeleton clearly confer advantages for different events and are almost entirely determined by genetic factors.

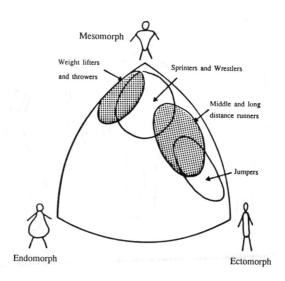

Fig. 5.12 Somatotypes and sporting ability. The three extreme somatotypes are shown together with the body types of different athletes (from Tanner, 1964).

It is not known why the biceps of a mesomorph is larger than that of an ectomorph. It could be that the muscle fibres grow to different sizes in the adult but, more likely, the mesomorph is born with more fibres, the number of myotubes that form the foetal muscle being genetically determined.

5.6 The use of anabolic drugs in sport

In the majority of mammals the male of the species tends to be larger and more heavily muscled than the female, the general belief being that the male is larger because he has higher levels of circulating testosterone (see also Section 5.4). It is this belief that has lead athletes, probably numbered in millions around the world, to possibly endanger their health by taking steroids, to become involved with illegal activities in order to obtain supplies and to risk the severe penalties imposed by the governing bodies of their sport.

Testosterone has two actions in the body, one, androgenic, is to stimulate the development of male secondary sexual characteristics, while the second is an anabolic function, promoting protein synthesis. In this latter role it is not clear whether the action is a direct effect of the hormone on the target organ or if it is first aromatised to oestradiol and acts via the secretion of GH. Much of the early interest in this subject was stimulated by the observation that testosterone caused an increase in size of the *levator ani* of castrated male rats, it being assumed that this was a good model for the action of testosterone on skeletal muscle in general. It is now clear that the rat *levator ani* is not a typical skeletal muscle as it forms part of the male reproductive tract in this animal. Properly controlled experiments have shown that body weight and lean body mass of the rat is little affected by testosterone in adult life, in fact high doses lead to a loss of weight. In rats, testosterone exerts its main effect very early in life when the high level of hormone during a short period after birth in the male determines the pattern of growth throughout life. Subsequent manipulation of the hormone levels has very little effect on growth patterns in rats (see Hervey, 1982).

The situation with the human male is confused. There are as many reports showing no change in skeletal muscle with administration of anabolic steroids as there are demonstrating increases in size or strength. The uncertainty arises partly because of the problems involved in organising effective trials. Quite apart from the ethical dilemma of giving a substance that may be harmful, the strict ban on the use of steroids makes it impossible for competitive athletes to openly participate. This is unfortunate because testosterone might prove to be of benefit only to certain somatotypes or to athletes who were prepared to undergo punishing training regimes, but without controlled trials it is impossible to make a rational judgement.

There is a general consensus that use of anabolic steroids can lead to an increase in body weight although there is doubt as to whether this is due to increased muscle or water. Where increased muscle has been demonstrated it appears to be of an abnormal composition, with more potassium and nitrogen than normal muscle (Hervey *et al*, 1981).

In addition to a possible effect of anabolic steroids increasing muscle protein synthesis, there are a number of other suggestions as to how testosterone might work in training. High doses lead to an increase in aggressive behaviour (androgenic action) which may be an advantage during training and competition. Alternatively, testosterone may help prevent, or speed recovery from, injury during training. This suggestion concerns the effects of cortisol which is produced in response to stress and reduces inflammatory responses and may promote healing. However cortisol also has a catabolic action on skeletal muscle (type 2 atrophy; see Chapter 11) and it has been suggested by Hervey (1982) that testosterone may block the catabolic action by competitive inhibition while allowing the healing actions to continue. At the same time testosterone might also slow the metabolism of cortisol in the liver, leading to higher circulating levels. Athletes taking anabolic steroids do have higher levels of cortisol and certainly report being able to train harder.

The risks of taking steroids are well known. With long-term use there is a possibility of liver damage and tumours developing. Anabolic steroids have the effect of feminising men and virilising women. This is because the preparations used have a low androgenic action yet still inhibit the secretion of GnRH from the hypothalamus. Consequently FSH and LH release is reduced and production of endogenous oestrogen and testosterone declines. The changes in secondary sexual characteristics and in fertility may be very slow to recover after stopping steroids. Use of steroids in very young athletes can have major effects altering both their physical and sexual development and is to be deplored. Although serious, the risks involved in taking anabolic steroids, at least for adult males, should be kept in proportion. This is especially so when compared to the harm which may be caused to bones, ligaments and tendons as a result of excessive "normal" training, not to mention the psychological and social cost of single-minded dedication to one activity.

Having discussed the physiological action of anabolic steroids the question must be asked: what improvements in competitive performance can be expected from taking steroids? A quantitative answer is very difficult to obtain, for the reasons outlined above, but one approach has been to plot world best performances year by year before and since the time when steroids came into use (Fig. 5.13). For the pole vault there was a clear step in performance when the glass-fibre pole was introduced, showing that this approach can detect significant advances in technique. If steroids conferred a clear benefit a similar step should be seen in events such as the discus and shot at about the time when anabolic steriods were first introduced. No significant improvement can be seen in these records and consequently the value of steroids for increasing performance remains unproven.

With improvements in the methods for detecting anabolic steroids in blood and urine, attention is beginning to move towards the possible use of GH, IGF1, GHRH or the basic amino acids which can cause release of GH. Detection of these substances is very difficult, if not impossible, since they have relatively short half times in the circulation and are also naturally occurring hormones or amino acids. *Human chorionic gonadotrophin* has also been used as it stimulates the natural production of testosterone, however, detection is relatively simple. A pregnancy test will give a very unexpected result for a male athlete who has been taking hCG since the standard pregnancy testing kits detect hCG.

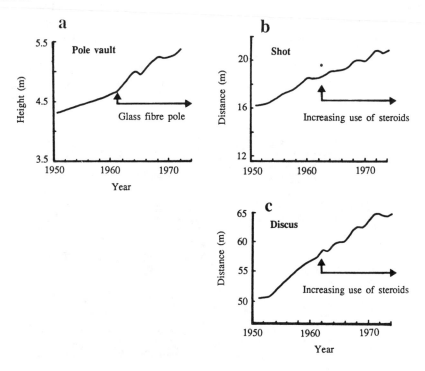

Fig. 5.13 World best performances. **a**, Pole vault showing the improvement with the introduction of the glass fibre pole in the early 1960s. **b** & **c**, Shot and discus; anabolic steroids have been increasingly used since the early 1960s (redrawn from Payne, 1975).

There is no reliable information as to whether these substances can increase muscle bulk in a normal adult or affect performance in any way. Excessive secretion of natural growth hormone causes acromegaly with large and distorted bones. The limited information about muscle function in acromegalic patients suggests that although large, their muscles are not particularly strong.

5.7 Ageing and muscle function

During and after the fifth decade there is a marked loss of muscle mass and a decrease in strength that is particularly notable in women when the hormonal balance is changed after the menopause. The loss is less severe in men below the age of about 70 years. The more rapid loss of muscle mass in women is reflected in a similar change in bone with women being much more susceptible to osteoporosis than men.

The loss of muscle in elderly subjects appears to be progressive and by the age of 90 years muscle mass can be reduced by 30%. The loss of muscle bulk is reported to be greater than can be accounted for by atrophy of the muscle fibres, indicating that fibre numbers may be reduced (Grimby & Saltin, 1983). It has been suggested that just as neuronal loss from the brain causes memory impairment in the elderly, so loss of motoneurones from the anterior horn causes a loss of motor units.

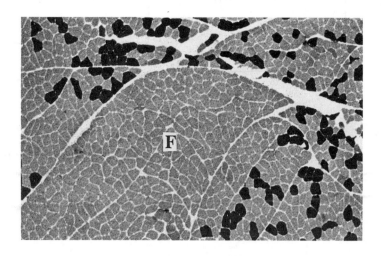

Fig. 5.14 Adductor pollicis muscle of the hand (autopsy sample, transverse section) from an elderly woman with no clinical neurological signs. F, fascicle containing only type 1 fibres indicating re-innervation (ATPase pH 9.4).

Histochemical examination of muscle specimens taken at autopsy from elderly subjects with no reported neurological symptoms frequently show areas of fibre type grouping suggesting some neurogenic disturbance has occurred (Fig. 5.14). These appearances could also be due to peripheral damage to motor nerves. It is of interest that the small muscles in the foot can show clear evidence of neuropathic change with increasing age which is thought to be a consequence of wearing shoes. Increased collagen cross-linking and lipofuchsin deposits in the muscle are also common findings. Whatever its cause, the loss of muscle may eventually becomes disabling so that subjects cannot rise from a chair or visit the toilet unaided. A decrease in mobility is an important cause of loss of independence and postponing its onset will become increasingly important as the number of elderly people surviving in the population increases. There is no evidence that habitual exercise can help to prevent the changes associated with ageing although, by preserving cardiac and respiratory function, regular exercise will help the elderly make the best use of the muscle that remains.

5.8 References and further reading

Brook, C.G.D. (ed.) (1989). *Clinical Paediatric Endocrinology*, 2nd edition, Oxford, Blackwell Scientific Publications.

Drager, A., Weeds, A.G. & Fitzsimons, R.B. (1987). Primary, secondary and tertiary myotubes in developing muscle: a new approach to the analysis of human myogenesis. *Journal of the Neurological Sciences* **81**, 19-43.

Faulkner, F. & Tanner, J.M. (ed.) (1985). *Human Growth: a Comprehensive Treatise.* New York, Plenum Press.

Florini, J.R. (1987). Hormonal control of muscle growth. *Muscle and Nerve* **10**, 577-98.

Grimby, G. & Saltin, B. (1983). The ageing muscle: a mini review. *Clinical Physiology* **3**, 209-18.

Hervey, G.R. (1982). What are the effects of anabolic steroids? In: *Science and Sporting Performance,* ed. B. Davies & G. Thomas. Oxford, Clarendon Press, pp. 120-360.

Hervey, G.R., Knibbs, A.V., Burkinshaw, L., Morgan, D.B., Jones, P.R.M., Chettle, D.R. & Vartsky, D. (1981). Effects of methandienone on the performance and body composition of men undergoing athletic training. *Clinical Science* **60**, 457-461.

Link, K., Blizzard, R.M., Evans, W.S., Kaiser, D.L., Parker, M.W. & Rogol, A.D. (1986). The effect of androgens on the pulsatile release and the twenty-four-hour mean concentration of growth hormone in peripubertal males. *Journal of Clinical Endocrinology and Metabolism* **62**, 159-64.

Payne, A.H. (1975). Anabolic steroids in athletics. *British Journal of Sports Medicine* **9**, 83-8.

Rowe, R.W.D. & Goldspink, G. (1969). Muscle fibre growth in five different muscles in both sexes of mice: I, normal mice. *Journal of Anatomy* **104**, 519-30.

Sheldon, W.H., Stevens, S.S. & Tucker, W.B. (1940). *Varieties of Human Physique.* New York, Harper.

Tanner, J.M. (1964). *The Physique of the Olympic Athlete.* London, George Allen & Unwin.

Chapter 6

TRAINING FOR POWER

The ingredients for success in all physical activities, whether of a sporting or more mundane everyday nature, are skill, strength, speed and endurance. The object of training is to match the mixture of ingredients to the requirements of the event and the deficiencies of the athlete. This chapter is concerned with training for the "explosive" events such as sprinting, jumping and throwing where the main concern is to maximise power output. Training for endurance events is dealt with in Chapter 7.

6.1 Definitions

Before beginning to discuss the merits of different training protocols, it is important briefly to consider what is meant by a number of commonly used words such as "force", "strength", "work" and "power".

Force is the most difficult word to define, mainly because forces, such as magnetic, electrostatic, gravitational, etc., cannot be seen. What can be seen and measured is the *effect* of a force. If a force is acting on an object it will begin to move and, if there is no opposing force such as friction, the mass will accelerate, moving faster and faster, so long as the force continues to act. Gravitational attraction is proportional to the mass of the body and, on the surface of the earth, it causes all objects to accelerate towards the centre at a rate of 9.81 metres/sec/sec. Thus if someone falls from a window they will be travelling at 9.81 metres/sec after one second of free fall and after the second second, at a speed of 19.62 metres/sec, providing there is no opposing force such as air resistance or the ground. By comparison, the gravitational pull on the surface of the moon is about one-ninth that of the earth's and the acceleration is therefore about one metre/sec/sec. In the real world, the reason why a cyclist or a sprinter does not continue to accelerate even though they may be applying continuous high forces to the pedals or to the running track, is that the resistance to movement builds up with the speed. The higher the velocity the higher the wind resistance and also the frictional resistance in the wheel bearings and, to a lesser extent, in the joints. Force is conventionally measured in Newtons (N) which is the force required to accelerate a mass of one Kg at one metre/sec/sec.

Since all objects fall towards the centre of the earth with an acceleration of 9.81 metre/sec/sec the gravitational force acting on a body to produce this acceleration must be 9.81 × the mass (weight) in kg. For the average 70 kg man, the force of gravity is 70 × 9.81 or about 700 N. It will therefore require a force of 700N to lift this average man off the ground. The words force and strength tend to be used interchangeably, strength being the ability to generate force.

When our average man climbs a flight of steps he will have done some work. The heavier he is and the higher he climbs, the more work he will have done. Work is the product of the force exerted and the distance through which it acts; the unit of measurement is the Joule (J). Our average man climbing a flight of stairs two metres high will have produced a force of 700N to lift himself off the ground and the work done will be 700N × 2 metres or 1400 J.

If we now had two average men who raced each other up the flight of steps, one taking one second, the other two seconds, both would have done the same amount of work, but the faster man would be the more powerful. Power is the rate of doing work and the unit of measurement is the Watt (W). Our fastest man will have done 1400 J in one second which is 1400 W. Our second man, having taken 2 seconds, will have had a power output of 700 W. Power is work divided by time (W = J/s = N × m/s). Velocity is distance divided by time (V = m/s) and so it can be seen that power can also be obtained by multiplying force by velocity (W = N × V).

6.2 Power output and performance

In sprinting events all competitors will do roughly the same amount of work, moving their own body weight (plus that of a bicycle if they are on wheels) against similar air and frictional resistances, over the same distance. The difference between the winner and loser is the time taken to do this work or, in other words, the power output. The object of training, therefore, must be to maximise power output during the competition. The power output of a muscle is determined by the velocity of shortening and the overall size and strength of the muscle.

When a muscle is stimulated it will attempt to shorten but if prevented from doing so will develop isometric force or tension. If the muscle is allowed to shorten the force that can be developed falls with increasing speed (Fig. 6.1) and eventually above a certain velocity, known as the maximum velocity of shortening (Vmax), the muscle can generate no force at all (see Chapter 2, Section 2.4.1). This behaviour can be understood by imagining a subject in a harness trying to pull as hard as possible while running on a treadmill. With the treadmill running slowly it is possible to pull quite hard but as the speed increases it becomes more difficult. When the treadmill reaches maximum sprinting speed the subject is being carried backwards as rapidly as he can run forward and it is impossible to exert any force on the harness. The maximum isometric force and Vmax are two important constants which characterise a muscle and determine the type of activity for which it is best suited.

The axes in Fig. 6.1 are force (y) and velocity (x) and force multiplied by velocity is power (see above). It is possible, therefore to calculate the power of a muscle and to see how this varies with velocity. It is also possible to see how power might be increased either by increasing Vmax or the maximum isometric force.

6.2.1 *Changes in maximum velocity of shortening*

If the maximum velocity of unloaded shortening of the muscle were to increase, the maximum power that could be obtained from the muscle would also increase (Fig. 6.1a).

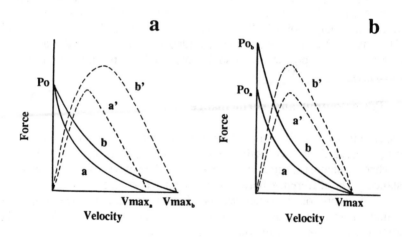

Fig. 6.1 Force/velocity relationships and possible changes with training. **a**, the effect of increasing maximum velocity of shortening (Vmaxa to Vmaxb). **b**, the effect of increasing maximum isometric force (Poa to Pob). Dashed line shows the power output, a' before, and b', after training.

The speed of a muscle depends on the proportions of the different types of fibre while the intrinsic velocity of shortening of an individual fibre is determined by the enzymic properties of the actomyosin cross-bridges. All muscle fibres contain the genetic information to express the different myosins and other proteins characteristic of fast and slow fibres, and it is therefore conceivable that the slow fibres might be induced to change into fast fibres as a result of training. Prolonged, relatively low force activity, such as that imposed by chronic low frequency electrical stimulation, causes a change to slow contractile characteristics (Chapter 4, Section 4.4). Evidence suggests, however, that a change from slow to fast characteristics does not occur as a result of training. Prolonged high frequency stimulation causes a slowing of contractile characteristics similar to that seen with low frequency stimulation and it seems unlikely that training will improve power output by increasing Vmax as a consequence of a change in gene expression. There is, however, another way of increasing shortening velocity. The velocity of shortening depends on the intrinsic speed of the muscle but is also proportional to its length (i.e. the number of sarcomeres in series along the fibre). If muscle length and sarcomere numbers can be increased, possibly as a result of stretching exercises, then the maximum velocity of shortening will be proportionately increased.

6.2.2 *Changes in strength*
If training is unlikely to increase the speed of shortening the only alternative, for those who wish to improve power output, is to try and increase the strength of the muscle.

Weight training is widely used as an adjunct to routine training for many sports, the general philosophy being that by increasing the size and strength of a specific muscle group, power output will be increased in events which use these muscles. This proves, however, to be a rather simplistic view.

By the early part of this century it had become apparent that muscle tends to increase in size as a result of performing work beyond its normal capacity (overload principle). In the 1950s and 1960s Hettinger & Müller carried out a series of experiments to determine the minimum stimulus required for an increase in muscle strength and the different factors such as age and sex that could affect trainability. They concentrated mainly on isometric exercise and concluded that one maximum isometric contraction of 1 to 2s duration a day was sufficient to produce maximum improvements in strength. In the course of their studies they noticed that there was a wide variation in the susceptibility of different subjects and muscles to training (Hettinger, 1961), a finding that continues to complicate all such investigations.

Since this early work, many studies have compared the effects of isometric, isokinetic and isotonic training with seemingly every combination of repetition number, number of training days a week and relative training loads (for review see McDonagh & Davies, 1984) but the basic conclusion that can be drawn is that as few as 10 repetitions a day at loads greater than 60 to 70% of maximum will, if carried out regularly, produce a small but steady increase in strength. However, the original claim of Hettinger & Müller that only one maximum contraction a day is sufficient has not been substantiated.

Despite the intense scientific and lay interest in strength training there remain many areas of ignorance and controversy. This chapter will deal mainly with three of these areas.

The first topic is the common observation that the benefits of training are very specific, being limited to the type of exercise undertaken and even to the speed of movement or the length of the active muscle.

The second is the question as to whether changes in strength are adequately explained by a change in size of the muscle: in other words, does training involve a change in quality as well as quantity of the muscle?

The final topic to be discussed concerns the nature of the stimulus for muscle hypertrophy. Despite the obvious importance of this topic, there is little evidence on which to base rational training regimes either for athletes and body builders or for patients undergoing rehabilitation following injury or illness.

6.3 Specificity of the training response

A common finding in the majority of studies on training is that the greatest changes accompanying strength training can be seen in the training exercise itself rather than in any objective assessment of muscle strength or size (for reviews see Sale & MacDougal, 1981; Jones *et al*, 1989).

6.3.1 *Task specificity*

There is an important difference between strength, defined as the ability to perform a task which may involve the coordinated contractions of a number of muscle groups, and the strength of an individual muscle. Training is frequently carried out by lifting weights in an apparatus such as a multi-gym and it is common experience that there will be a much greater increase in the ability to lift weights than in the intrinsic strength of the muscle groups being trained.

One of the early indications that training is specific to the movement pattern was reported by Rasch & Morehouse (1957). Subjects trained the elbow flexors in the standing position and were subsequently assessed both standing and supine. The increase in muscle strength was much greater in the familiar than in the unfamiliar position. A further indication of the specificity of movement pattern comes from studies examining changes in power output accompanying strength training. In one study, subjects trained for 12 weeks by lifting near maximal loads on a leg extension machine (Rutherford *et al*, 1986). After three months of training, the improvement in training load was of the order of 200% accompanied by only a 15% increase in the isometric strength of the quadriceps (Fig. 6.2).

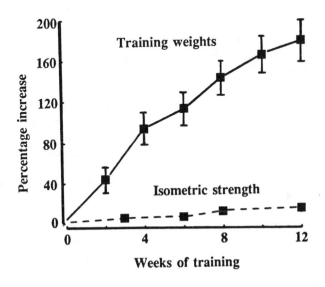

Fig. 6.2 Changes of strength with training. Changes in weights lifted during training compared with the gain in isometric strength of the quadriceps muscles.

The performance of a different task, maximum power output measured on a cycle ergometer, showed no change over the twelve weeks. Thus despite the improvement in the familiar training manoeuvre there was no significant change in power output measured in an unfamiliar manner, although the quadriceps was one of the main muscle groups involved in both the training and in isokinetic cycling. Such a lack of cross-over in performance suggests that the large increase in training weights lifted may be attributable to acquisition of skill in the training task, lifting weights, which was of little value in the different task of riding a bicycle.

Task specificity may be accounted for by an improvement in coordination of the different muscle groups that are involved in activities such as learning to ride a bicycle or write with the non- dominant hand. The neural pathways involved in such learning are clearly complex, may exist at several levels in the central nervous system and involve various sensory inputs from skin, joints, eyes and the vestibular system. Although superficially many tasks appear to require minimal skill this is only because these skills have been unconsciously acquired during childhood. Watching subjects make maximal contractions it is immediately obvious that they are also contracting many different muscles to stabilise the particular limb and the rest of the body. Contraction of abdominal and chest wall muscles seems to be a universal and necessary response to making a large effort and is part of the skill that has to be acquired.

Most people have a dominant side and can throw a ball nearly twice as far with this arm compared to the non-dominant side. We tend to say that one arm is stronger than the other, but in most people there is little more than a 5 or 10% difference in strength of individual muscles on the two sides. The difference lies in the ability to coordinate the correct sequence of muscle contractions. If, as a result of injury, a person is forced to use their non-dominant limb they can, in time, learn to do so very effectively. The message here is that when it comes to complex tasks the strength of any particular muscle is only one of the factors contributing to performance; without the necessary skill and coordination a strong muscle is of little value.

6.3.2 *Length and velocity specificity*

There is some evidence that if training is carried out at a fixed muscle length or a specific speed of contraction then the benefits are seen only at that particular speed or length. Superficially this seems an unlikely adaptation for muscle since these changes imply an alteration in the form of the length-tension or force-velocity relationships, both of which are fundamental properties of the myofilaments, and it would be difficult to explain how a bump could appear in either of these curves. However the observations of specificity have been made on whole muscle groups using voluntary contractions. In the case of length specificity it is possible that preferential hypertrophy of one of the constituent muscle groups might change the relationship of the whole muscle (Fig. 6.3). Likewise a change in length of the muscle might also appear to lead to greater increases in force at either short or long length compared to a mid length position.

The evidence for velocity specificity is far from convincing as measurements of force-velocity properties are difficult to make in large muscle groups such as the quadriceps.

Changes in fibre type composition in a mixed muscle might lead to a change in the force-velocity curves and, again, a change in overall length would lead to a greater maximum velocity which would lead to greater proportional changes in strength at the high velocities (Fig. 6.1a).

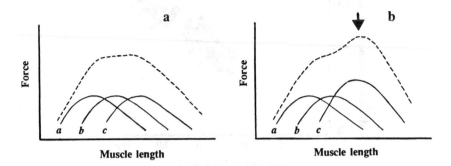

Fig. 6.3 The effect of selective hypertrophy on the length-tension relationship of a compound muscle group. The group is made up of three muscles, *a, b* & *c* which have overlapping curves which combine to give the relationship shown as the dashed line. **a**, before training. **b**, after training the effect of hypertrophy of muscle *c* is a change in the relationship of the whole muscle.

Specificity of any description is widely attributed to "neural adaptation". It is possible that in the untrained state subjects are not able, by voluntary effort, to fully activate muscle groups at certain speeds or with the limb held in certain positions. There is no doubt that during rapid movements it is difficult for the subject to be sure that the effort is truly maximal and contractions certainly feel very unusual when holding an arm or leg in a fully flexed or extended position. Training may help the subject to fully activate the muscle over the full range of movement and speeds but at present the little evidence there is suggests that most subjects are able to fully activate their quadriceps muscles in most situations.

6.4 Changes in muscle strength and size during training

The major determinant of strength is muscle size, or more specifically, the cross-sectional area (CSA). About 50% of the variation in strength between people can be explained by differences in muscle size (Fig. 6.4) and it is important to establish whether it is increases in size or some other factor that accounts for the improvements in strength with training.

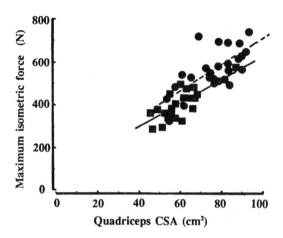

Fig. 6.4 Muscle cross-sectional area and strength. CSA of the quadriceps measured by CT scanning; results for young men (●) and women (■). The regressions have r values of approximately 0.75, indicating that about 50% of the variation is explained by differences in CSA.

A number of short-term training studies have demonstrated increases in strength that are greater than increases in muscle size (Fig. 6.5). Once again the explanations for this phenomenon have centred on "neural adaptations" although there are also several peripheral mechanisms which could result in an increased force per unit area.

6.4.1 *Neural mechanisms*

It has been suggested that prior to training muscle cannot be maximally activated by voluntary activity, and that in the first 6-8 weeks of training, before changes in muscle size become apparent, activation, and therefore strength, increases as a result of altered neural drive.

There are two main ways in which neural adaptation could result in an increase in the maximum voluntary isometric strength.

1. Large, fast, motor units are recruited only at higher forces and it has been suggested that during maximal voluntary contractions there are some units that are never recruited in the untrained state. Training is therefore seen as a way of facilitating the recruitment of these large and fast motor units.

2. It is possible that changes occur in the pattern of electrical stimulation of motor units, either by an increase in the firing frequency or in the synchronisation of firing between motor units. These two changes should be evident in the electrical activity of the trained muscle ˙ but there are considerable technical problems associated with monitoring EMG activity over a prolonged training period. The EMG signal picked up from surface electrodes is critically dependent on their position on the

skin relative to the muscle and on the impedance of the skin and underlying tissues. With care it is probably possible to relocate the electrodes with reasonable accuracy and most investigators go to some lengths to prepare the skin and reduce skin resistance to a low and constant value. What is not possible to control is the subcutaneous and intramuscular fat content which may vary over the course of a prolonged training study. Komi (1986) has summarised the evidence that in trained muscle there is an increase in synchronisation of motor unit firing. It is not clear how this change would give rise to an increase in isometric strength but it could be functionally important then it is necessary to coordinate a rapid series of movements such as are required during jumping or throwing.

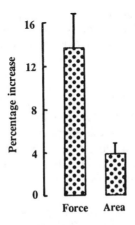

Fig. 6.5 Changes in muscle size and strength as a result of training. Quadriceps CSA and strength measured before and after 12 weeks training (see Fig. 6.2). Note the strength gain is larger than the change in size.

6.4.2 Peripheral mechanisms

A different approach to the question of whether a muscle is fully activated is to stimulate the voluntarily contracting muscle to see whether any additional force can be obtained (Merton, 1954; Fig. 6.6). The general conclusion from this type of investigation is that most normal subjects can fully activate most muscle groups without any training (Jones & Rutherford, 1987).

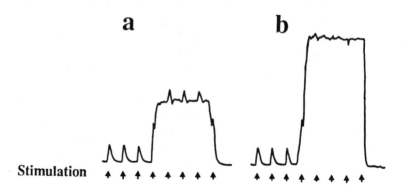

Fig. 6.6 Electrical stimulation superimposed on voluntary contractions. The muscle was stimulated with single twitches (arrows) while the subject made either submaximal (a) or maximal (b) contractions. During the maximal contraction there was no additional force on stimulation.

Alternative explanations for the discrepancy between changes in muscle strength and size following training concern possible alterations in the composition of the muscle. In addition to the CSA of the muscle other factors which may affect strength include the lever system through which strength is measured, fibre type composition, fibre architecture and the packing of contractile material. It is conceivable that the last three could be modified by a period of strength training.

6.4.2.1 *Fibre type composition* There is some evidence from both human and animal work that type 2 fibres are intrinsically stronger than type 1. Preferential type 2 hypertrophy or an increased type 2 frequency after training would lead to a greater increase in muscle strength compared to CSA in a mixed muscle. Although elite power athletes have ben found to have large type 2 fibres the evidence for preferential hypertrophy or change in frequency in short term training studies is contradictory (Rutherford, 1988). Where selective hypertrophy has been found, the differences have been too small to account for the disparity between changes in strength and size. Neither is there any evidence for fibre type conversion after strength training regimes (for review see Edström & Grimby, 1986).

6.4.2.2 *The angle of muscle fibre insertion* Individual muscles vary in the arrangement of their fibres between tendons (see Fig. 1.2), the simplest architecture being when the fibres lie parallel to the line of action of the muscle (parallel muscle). Many muscles, including the four portions of the quadriceps are pennate, that is, the fibres insert into the tendons at acute angles. A change in this angle of insertion (or pennation) may alter the force measured between the ends of a muscle. For the same length and anatomical CSA of muscle an increased angle of pennation can result in more contractile material being attached to a larger area of tendon (Alexander & Vernon, 1975). If, as a result of training, there was a simultaneous increase in both the angle at which fibres attach to the tendon and their CSA, then, with a small reduction in fibre length, the overall change in muscle CSA would be smaller than that in fibre area.

6.4.2.3 *Contractile material packing* An increase in force per unit area could be explained by an increased packing of the contractile material. This could involve either a closer packing of the actin and myosin or a loss of fat and connective tissue from between the fibres. There is little evidence for an increase in myofilament packing nor any firm data about changes in fat content with training.

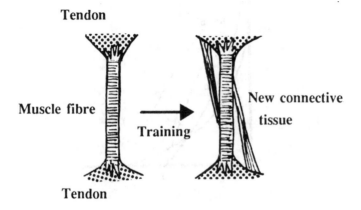

Fig. 6.7 Changes in connective tissue leading to an increase in force. The possible formation of links between tendon and intermediate points on the fibre leads to an increase in force but a reduction in effective fibre length.

6.4.2.4 *Connective tissue attachments* It is generally assumed that tension is transmitted longitudinally in a muscle fibre through serial sarcomeres so that the force is proportional only to the CSA and independent of the length. If, however, attachments were made between the tendons and intermediate sarcomeres this would increase the force generated per unit CSA of muscle (Fig. 6.7).

Mammalian muscle fibres are enveloped in a connective tissue matrix which could play some role in transmitting tension to the tendons. Work-induced hypertrophy is known to increase collagen synthesis in animal muscle and the increased radiological density found after training in humans could result from an increased connective tissue content.

6.4.2.5   *Consequences for power output*   Changes in the muscle
architecture or in the connective tissue attachments to the muscle fibres
resulting in a greater isometric force will also reduce the effective length
of the muscle fibres.   The change might be an absolute loss of fibre
length with change in pennation or, where connective tissue attachments
are made at points along the fibre, there could be a reduction in the
functional muscle length.   In either case, the loss of length would be
expected to result in a lower maximum velocity of shortening because
there would be fewer sarcomeres in series along the line of action of the
muscle.

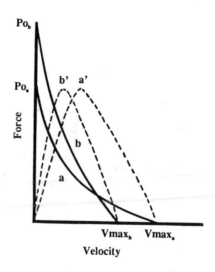

Fig. 6.8   Consequences of increased connective tissue. a, before training, b, after
changes leading to an increase in Po_a to Po_b and decrease in $Vmax_a$ to $Vmax_b$. Dashed
lines show power output before a' and after, b' training.

The combination of an increased isometric force and decreased
velocity of shortening would result in variable changes in power output
depending upon the velocity at which the measurement was made.   At
low velocities the trained muscle would be expected to be more
powerful, although the percentage increase would not be as great as for
the isometric force alone, while at higher velocities of shortening the
trained muscle would be less powerful (Fig. 6.8).

The velocity at which the maximum power output was achieved
would be expected to decrease if there was a shortening of the effective
muscle length.   To date there is little experimental evidence to test these
ideas.

6.5 The stimulus for increase in strength

A great deal has been written about the merits of different training protocols and it is of obvious importance to establish the most effective means of increasing strength. The general consensus is that high forces have to be employed before any new muscle growth is obtained. However, it is not clear whether it is the high force *per se* that is the stimulus for change or simply that it is a means of ensuring that all motor units are recruited and subjected to a training stimulus such as the large metabolic changes associated with heavy exercise.

All growth requires the remodelling of existing structures, i.e. an increased turnover involving both synthesis and degradation, but an increase in tissue size implies an excess of protein synthesis over protein degradation.   There are two aspects to protein turnover, one a maintenance of some basal tissue size for which turnover needs to respond to short term changes in glucose, amino acids and hormones such as insulin.   Control at this level is probably at the translational level with fluctuations in the "RNA activity".   The second aspect of control occurs over a longer time scale. The laying down of more tissue is probably dependent upon increased ribosomal content which, in turn, may require division of satellite cells and incorporation of one of the daughter nuclei into the muscle fibre.   In this way the nuclear material increases and the DNA unit size (the ratio of protein to DNA in the muscle) remains constant (Waterlow *et al*, 1978).

The possible stimuli for muscle hypertrophy can be divided into three categories:

6.5.1 *Hormonal stimuli*

Exercise may result in endocrine or paracrine responses that stimulate muscle growth.   It is unlikely that endocrine changes are the major stimulus since hypertrophy can be limited to a single muscle group on one side of the body but paracrine responses (local production of growth factors) may be important.

6.5.2 *Metabolic stimuli*

Most people training with weights instinctively feel that "it has to hurt to do any good".   The hurting referred to is the burning sensation associated with metabolic changes in the working muscles.   Despite this common sentiment there is no clear indication as to whether metabolic depletion is a prerequisite for change.   Heavy exercise will result in large metabolic fluxes in the tissue with the accumulation of high concentrations of H^+, inorganic phosphate and creatine, together with smaller quantities of other substances such as ADP, NH_3 and inosine, and it is possible that one or more of these metabolites could stimulate muscle growth. However, these metabolite changes are associated with fatiguing rather than strengthening exercises and it is more likely that they would be a stimulus for the mitochondrial proliferation and capillary growth, associated with increased endurance, rather than an increase in muscle size and strength. In conditions where there is an impaired oxygen supply to a muscle and metabolites are likely to be chronically in a depleted state, such as with peripheral vascular disease, the adaptation which occurs is an increase in the mitochondrial content rather then an increase in size. Highly trained endurance athletes do not have muscles that are especially strong.

Training exercises in which muscles are stretched (eccentric exercise or negative work) can generate forces in the active muscles that are considerably greater than the more conventional exercise in which muscles shorten as weights are lifted. In addition, because in eccentric exercise work is absorbed rather than generated by the muscle, the metabolic cost for a given force generated are far less than during concentric work (Bigland-Ritchie & Woods, 1976). A comparison of training using eccentric or concentric contractions should therefore provide a means of testing whether the stimulus for muscle growth is high force or metabolite changes. However the majority of studies which have used this approach have not shown a difference between the two types of exercise (Jones & Rutherford, 1987) and the relative importance of force and metabolic change remains unresolved.

6.5.3 *Mechanical factors*

It is well established that muscles held in shortened or lengthened positions rapidly change their overall length so that the sarcomere lengths are restored to something like the optimum for force generation (Williams & Goldspink, 1978). This is achieved by addition or removal of sarcomeres from the ends of the fibres. As well as affecting the length, stretching muscle appears to cause muscular hypertrophy (Laurent *et al*, 1978).

There are a number of ways in which muscle turnover might be affected by mechanical stress.

1. High force can cause micro damage to the sarcomere structure and thereby provide a stimulus for repair and compensatory growth. Goldspink (1971) has suggested that high forces lead to disruption of the Z disks causing the myofibril to split, the fragments then growing back to full size (Fig. 6.9). This is an attractive visual model and dislocations of Z lines can be seen in EM photographs especially after exercise involving high force eccentric contractions (Fridén *et al*, 1983).

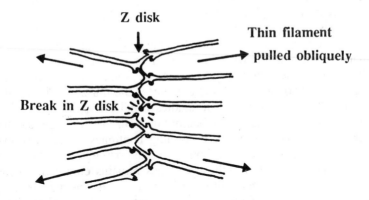

Fig. 6.9 Mechanism whereby myofibrils may increase in number with training. In large myofibrils the oblique pull of the thin filaments on the Z disk causes a tear and creation of two smaller myofibrils which can regrow to the original size (redrawn from Goldspink, 1971).

2.   Using isolated preparations of rat diaphragm or rabbit skeletal muscle, Reeds *et al* (1987) have shown that mechanical stimulation (repeated stretching of the resting muscle) causes an increase in both protein synthesis and degradation and they suggest that the activity activates phospholipases which liberate aracidonic acid which is the precursor for prostaglandin synthesis. It would be interesting to know whether body builders need to avoid taking too many aspirins since aspirin is a cylo-oxygenase inhibitor which prevents the formation of prostaglandins.
3.   Connective tissue: The connective tissue network is an integral part of muscle and must grow and change with the muscle fibres.   The connective tissue matrix also provides the connection between the force generating components and the tendons and, as such, will be subject to mechanical stress. It is possible that fibroblasts in the connective tissue might produce growth factors such as IGF1 (see Chapter 5, Section 5.3.3) in response to mechanical stress.

6.6 Summary

The picture of training for power that emerges is of a progressive change that can be divided into a number of phases. In the first phase there is a rapid improvement in the ability to perform a training exercise such as lifting weights, the improvement being the result of a learning process in which the correct sequence of muscle contractions is laid down as a motor pattern in the central nervous system. This phase is associated with little or no increase in the size or strength of individual muscles. The learning process appears to be very specific in that lifting weights makes better weight lifters but not better sprinters or jumpers. The second phase is an increase in the strength of individual muscles which occurs without a matching increase in the anatomical cross section. The mechanism for this increase in strength is not clear but it could be a result of increased neural activation or some change in the fibre arrangement or connective tissue content of the muscle. The third phase starts at a point where scientific studies usually end, at about 12 weeks when non-athletic subjects are beginning to tire of the repeated training and testing. After this point, if training continues, there is probably a slow but steady increase in both size and strength of the exercised muscles. The stimulus for these changes remains enigmatic but almost certainly involves the generation of high forces in the muscle, probably to induce some form of damage that promotes division of satellite cells and their incorporation into existing muscle fibres. Despite considerable interest in the subject there is still very little understanding of the underlying mechanisms controlling muscle growth on which to base training programmes to increase strength and power output.

6.7 References and further reading

Alexander, R. McN. & Vernon, A. (1975). The dimensions of the knee and ankle muscles and the forces they exert. *Journal of Human Movement Studies* **1**, 115-23.

Bigland-Ritchie, B. & Woods, J.J. (1976). Integrated electromyograms and oxygen uptake during positive and negative work. *Journal of Physiology* **260**, 267-77.

Edström, L. & Grimby, L. (1986). Effect of exercise on the motor unit. *Muscle & Nerve* **9**, 104-26.

Fridén, J., Sjöstrom, M. & Ekblom, B. (1983). Myofibrillar damage following intense eccentric exercise in man. *International Journal of Sports Medicine* **4**, 170-6.

Goldspink, G. (1971). Ultrastructural changes in striated muscle fibres during contraction and growth with particular reference to the mechanism of myofibril splitting. *Journal of Cell Science* **9**, 123-38.

Hettinger, T. (1961). *Physiology of Strength.* Springfield, C.C. Thomas.

Jones, D.A. & Rutherford, O.M. (1987). Human muscle strength training: the effects of three different training regimes and the nature of the resultant changes. *Journal of Physiology* **391**, 1-11.

Jones, D.A., Rutherford, O.M. & Parker, D.F. (1989). Physiological changes in skeletal muscle as a result of strength training. *Quarterly Journal of Experimental Physiology* **74**, 233-56.

Komi, P.V. (1986). How important is neural drive for strength and power development in human skeletal muscle? In: *Biochemistry of Exercise VI* ed. B. Saltin. International Series on Sport Sciences, Vol. 16. Champaign, Ill. Human Kinetics Publishers, pp. 515-29.

Laurent, G.J., Sparrow, M.P. & Millward, D.J. (1978). Turnover of muscle protein in the fowl. Changes in rates of protein synthesis and breakdown during hypertrophy of the anterior and posterior latissimus dorsi muscles. *Biochemical Journal* **176**, 407-17.

McDonagh, M.J.N. & Davies, C.T.M. (1984). Adaptive response of mammalian skeletal muscle to exercise with high loads. *European Journal of Applied Physiology* **52**, 139-55.

Merton, P.A. (1954). Voluntary strength and fatigue. *Journal of Physiology* **123**, 553-64.

Rasch, P.J. & Morehouse, L.E. (1957). Effect of static and dynamic exercises on muscular strength and hypertrophy. *Journal of Applied Physiology* **11**, 29-34.

Reeds, P.J., Palmer, R.M. & Wahle, K.W.J. (1987). The role of metabolites of arachidonic acid in the physiology and pathophysiology of muscle protein metabolism. *Biochemical Society Transactions* **15**, 328-31.

Rutherford, O.M. (1988). Muscular coordination and strength training: implications for injury rehabilitation. *Sports Medicine* **5**, 196-202.

Rutherford, O.M., Greig, C.A., Sargaent, A.J. & Jones, D.A. (1986). Strength training and power output: transference effects in the human quadriceps muscle. *Journal of Sports Science* **4**, 101-7.

Sale, D.G. & MacDougall, J.D. (1981). Specificity in strength training; a review for the coach and athlete. *Canadian Journal of Applied Sports Science* **6**, 87-92.

Waterlow, J.C., Garlick, P.J. & Millward, D.J. (1978). *Protein Turnover in Mammalian Tissues and in the Whole Body*. Amsterdam, North Holland.

Williams, P. & Goldspink, G. (1978). Changes in sarcomere length and physiological properties in immobilized muscle. *Journal of Anatomy* **127**, 459-68.

Chapter 7

ADAPTATIONS FOR ENDURANCE EXERCISE

Endurance essentially means avoiding the effects of fatigue. Changes that lead to a loss of performance, or fatigue, can be grouped broadly into *central* and *peripheral* factors. A decrease in central drive may occur as a result of hypoglycaemia, increase in core temperature or pain originating in peripheral tissues under stress. Peripheral factors are changes in muscle function as a consequence of metabolic depletion or damage. Fatigue is dealt with more fully in Chapter 8 but the main features relevant to training are summarised here in Sections 7.1 and 7.2.

7.1 Central drive

A loss of central drive (central fatigue) can include a wide range of changes in the central nervous system, some of which may impinge on the consciousness as pain and discomfort. Others, such as reflex changes in motoneurone firing, may be quite unconscious. The discomforts of prolonged exercise are familiar and include the sensations of breathlessness, raised core temperature and pain in joints and working muscles. These sensations are enough to persuade most people to ease up but, with training, the discomforts are tolerated better. This is partly due to physiological adaptations such as greater oxidative capacity and better temperature regulation reducing the acidosis or core temperature for a given level of work. However, there may also be central adaptations in the perception of the noxious stimuli. Trained athletes can exercise for prolonged periods with ventilation rates comparable to, or higher than, those which can be tolerated by untrained subjects and they can also tolerate greater acidosis than inexperienced subjects. Exercise can cause the release of endorphins (naturally occurring peptides with opioid activity) and these substances may help to "anaesthetize" the athlete to the discomfort. Whatever the mechanism, training leads to a reduction in the central distress associated with exercise and in so doing may reduce central fatigue. Although not always obvious, endurance events involve an element of skill, which, as with the improvements in coordination discussed in the previous chapter, can be improved with training. An efficient running style is very important to conserve energy in long distance races and entails good balance and elimination of unnecessary movements of the arms or head. Loss of running style is often an indication of the onset of fatigue.

Despite the importance of central drive, the neurological and psychological factors involved are difficult to identify and quantitate so that most attention in endurance training has focused on physiological adaptations of the respiratory and cardiovascular systems together with changes in skeletal muscle function.

7.2 Peripheral fatigue

Peripheral mechanisms of fatigue are complex and poorly understood but there is no doubt that metabolic depletion plays an important role in reducing muscle function; the uncertainty arises in knowing which is the key metabolite and the mechanism whereby force is decreased (see Chapter 8).

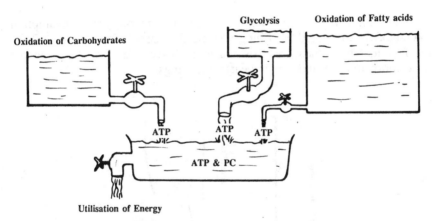

Fig. 7.1 The balance between supply and demand for energy during exercise. Note that the rate of supply differs for the various substrates and the larger the reserve the slower the supply; PC, phosphocreatine.

Glycolysis alone can supply energy for only a limited time so that for any endurance exercise the body is dependent on oxidative metabolism to maintain the necessary level of ATP. The "water running into a bath" model (Fig. 7.1) illustrates the essentials of muscle energetics with respect to exercise. If the rate at which water runs out of a bath is greater than the rate of entry, the water level (energy reserves) will fall. The immediate energy reserves are ATP and phosphocreatine and, as the reserves fall below some crucial level, muscle function deteriorates so that endurance (the length of time the subject can work at a given power output) is determined by the balance between the rates of provision and utilization of ATP.

7.3 Energy supply

The provision of energy for any exercise lasting more than a minute or so is limited by the rate of supply of oxygen to the tissue, the availability of fuels for oxidation, mitochondria and the appropriate enzymes.

7.3.1 *Supply of oxygen*
The supply of oxygen to the tissues may be divided into three areas of interest: ventilation and gas exchange at the lungs, the cardiac output and peripheral circulation which determines the amount of oxygen delivered to the tissue and, lastly, diffusion into the cells and the capacity of the tissue to utilise oxygen.

7.3.1.1   *The lungs*   Although the maximum oxygen consumption (VO$_2$max) is correlated with lung volume this association mainly reflects the fact that both measures are related to body size since large people have more muscle and larger hearts and lungs.

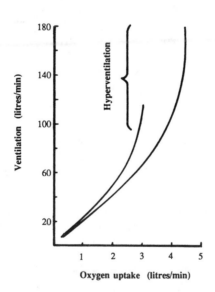

Fig. 7.2 Pulmonary ventilation and oxygen uptake at different levels of exercise. Results are shown for two subjects with differing VO$_2$max. Note the phase of hyperventilation towards the end of the exercise.

There is circumstantial evidence that lung mechanics do not limit exercise in normal subjects. Towards the end of a progressive exercise test, during which the workload is increased in steps every few minutes, there is a phase of hyperventilation (Fig. 7.2). At this stage the volume of gas passing in and out of the lungs continues to increase but the body is unable to use any more oxygen indicating that lung mechanics and ventilation are not the factors that limit the exercise. It is doubtful whether endurance training increases lung volume although there are suggestions that training during childhood and adolescence may result in larger volumes in the adult.

Diffusion of gas in the alveoli is probably not a limiting factor. CO_2 diffusion is very rapid but although oxygen equilibrates more slowly, in the majority of normal subjects oxygen saturation in the arterial blood remains constant and high (>90%) throughout exercise. Only in exceptional athletes does desaturation of the arterial blood occur at the highest levels of exercise.

7.3.1.2 *Cardiovascular factors* A large cardiac output is associated with high VO_2max. Trained endurance athletes have hearts that are appreciably larger than normal for their body size (Fig. 7.3). Cardiac stroke volume is increased in these people but there is probably not a large increase in left ventricular wall thickness. Training can lead to an increase in cardiac output of about 20%, the precise value depending very much on the level of habitual activity before the training. Increased stroke volume is accompanied by a reduction in heart rate at rest and during submaximal exercise and a greater cardiac output at maximum heart rate.

Other things being equal, the ability to transport oxygen will be limited by the haemoglobin content of the blood. However, endurance trained athletes have normal or even slightly low haemoglobin concentrations, possibly as a result of increased mechanical damage to red cells during running. Training at altitude increases the numbers of red cells in circulation and, thereby, the total haemoglobin content. A similar improvement can be achieved by the practice of "blood doping" in which blood is withdrawn and then, several weeks later when the numbers of red cells have returned to normal, reinfused just before a race to give an increased haemoglobin content (Thomson *et al*, 1982). There are probably limits to the value of this latter activity as an increase in blood viscosity could be counterproductive, increasing peripheral resistance. Two, three- diphosphoglycerate (2,3-DPG), formed in red blood cells in active tissues, shifts the haemoglobin dissociation curve to the left, facilitating oxygen uptake by the tissue. 2,3-DPG production is reported to be increased in red blood cells as a result of training.

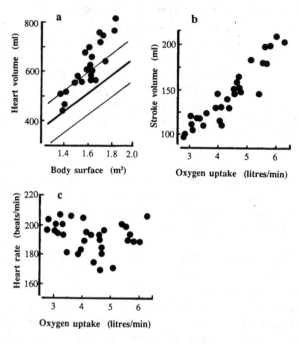

Fig. 7.3 Heart size and cardiac output in relation to maximum oxidative work capacity. **a**, heart volume in relation to body size (surface area) in the general population (lines giving mean and range) compared to trained athletes, individual points (redrawn from Åstrand *et al*, 1963). **b**, stroke volume and VO₂max in a wide range of trained and untrained subjects. **c**, heart rate and VO₂max in subjects shown in **b** (redrawn from Ekblom, 1969).

An increase in capillary density in skeletal muscle is one of the first changes to occur during endurance training; trained subjects may have 30% more capillaries than untrained. The slow oxidative type 1 fibres generally have a higher capillary density, about 3 to 4 per fibre as opposed to 2 to 3 for the type 2 fibres, and the proximity of capillaries to the fibre improves the diffusion of oxygen. The physical stimulus of increased blood flow at the bends of small capillaries probably causes sprouting and the formation of an extended capillary bed in skeletal and cardiac muscle (Hudlicka, 1988).

Other factors that improve diffusion are the size of the muscle fibres and their myoglobin content. Endurance trained athletes tend to have muscles which are somewhat smaller than the average because their muscle fibres are smaller in cross-section. The advantage of this is that diffusion distances for oxygen are reduced. Patterns of artificial electrical stimulation of muscles in man and animals leading to an improvement in fatigue resistance also result in a reduction in muscle force, probably because the muscle fibres become smaller. The myoglobin content of slow fibres is higher than in fast fibres and functions to facilitate oxygen diffusion from the capillary into the fibres. The rate of diffusion is approximately doubled by the presence of myoglobin. In diving mammals myoglobin acts as an oxygen store but in man its main function is probably to assist diffusion. Myoglobin content of muscle probably increases with endurance training but there is little information on this topic.

The other major factor limiting utilisation of oxygen is the number of mitochondria in a muscle; this can change markedly with training and is discussed in Section 7.3.3 below.

7.3.2 Supply of fuel

The two major fuels used by muscle are carbohydrate, in the form of glucose or glycosyl units, and free fatty acids. Oxidation of amino acids makes only a minor contribution to the provision of energy during exercise. The carbohydrate and fatty acids either arrive at the muscle in the blood having been released from liver or adipose tissue, or are obtained from intracellular stores of glycogen and triglyceride within the muscle fibre (Fig. 7.4).

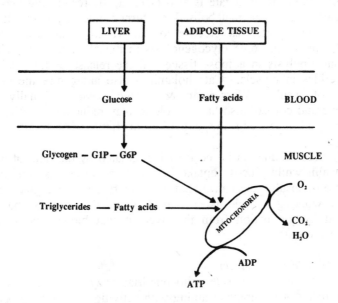

Fig. 7.4 Energy sources available for oxidative metabolism during exercise.

During exercise there are a number of hormonal changes, the effect of which is to provide skeletal muscle with sufficient substrate while ensuring that the active muscle does not deplete the blood of glucose, causing hypoglycaemia with attendant central complications. The changes are summarised in Table 7.1; the decrease in insulin has the effect of stopping glucose uptake by adipose tissue and minimising uptake by the active muscle.

INCREASE	DECREASE
Adrenaline	Insulin
Noradrenaline	
Glucagon	
ACTH	
Cortisol	
Growth hormone	

Table 7.1   Hormonal changes during prolonged exercise.

Glucagon causes the release of glucose from the liver and also stimulates gluconeogenesis, the liver using lactate from the working muscles. Circulating lactate is also taken up by resting muscles and by the heart and either metabolised or turned into glycogen; it is not, however, re-exported as glucose to the working muscles. Increased catecholamines promote glycogenolysis in muscle and liver. They also stimulate lipolysis in adipose tissue and the release of fatty acids from triglycerides in muscle. Catecholamines also antagonise the peripheral effects of insulin (Wasserman & Vranic, 1986). Finally, growth hormone and cortisol also have a role to play reducing the utilization of glucose and increasing the oxidation of fatty acids by the working muscle.

Glucose production in the liver is regulated by the ratio of glucagon and insulin while glucose uptake in peripheral tissues is determined by the ratio of insulin and catecholamines. During exercise glucose uptake by the working muscle is increased about three times, but this is matched by production from the liver so that blood glucose remains relatively constant.

7.3.3   *Muscle composition*

An increase in muscle mitochondrial enzyme content is a well-known result of endurance training with activities of many mitochondrial enzymes increasing two to threefold. Muscle biopsies from highly trained subjects show an abundance of mitochondria, often accumulating just beneath the sarcolemma, but it is not clear whether the increased enzyme activity is entirely explained by the increased mitochondrial volume or whether there has also been a qualitative change. High VO_2max is generally associated with high mitochondrial activities although there is not a clear correlation between enzyme levels and oxygen uptake.

The high capillary density, myoglobin and mitochondrial content of the trained muscle have obvious advantages for endurance exercise and can occur as the result of adaptation to prolonged endurance training in muscles of any fibre composition. The thigh muscles of top class marathon runners are generally composed of predominantly (about 70%) type 1, slow oxidative fibres (Fig. 7.5) which have high oxidative capacity even in the untrained state.

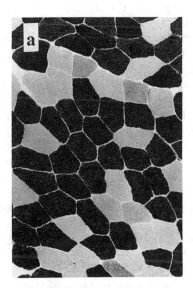 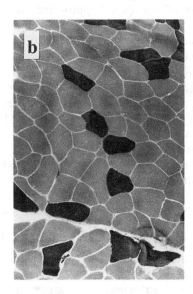

Fig. 7.5 Fibre type composition of the quadriceps in athletes. **a**, high jumper. **b**, quality marathon runner. Myosin ATPase, pH 9.4; the type 2 fibres stain dark.

The predominance of slow fibres raises an interesting question as to whether the top class marathon runners are born with their complement of slow fibres or have acquired them as a result of years of intense training. Prolonged activity, imposed by electrical stimulation in animals, will change the fibre type composition of a muscle (Chapter 4, Section 4.4) but expression of myosin isoenzymes is one of the last characteristics to change and there is some doubt as to whether voluntary activity, even running 100 miles a week, could provide a sufficient stimulus for change. Running on the level at marathon pace probably only requires about 20% of the maximum quadriceps contraction and this would involve the recruitment of only the slow motor units. It is not clear, therefore, how the large, fast units would receive their training stimulus. Studies with identical twins show that there is a strong genetic component determining the fibre type composition of muscle, as there is for VO_2max and it seems likely that top class marathon runners may be genetically endowed with a high proportion of type 1 fibres. This question will only be settled by a longitudinal study of changes in muscle fibre composition with training, but the practical difficulties of such a study are formidable. A more feasible study might be to follow changes in top class marathon runners who had given up training to see whether their unusual fibre type composition persisted. Unfortunately for physiology (but happily for the life style of the athletes), top class endurance runners enjoy running and do not suddenly retire into inactivity but tend gradually to decrease their level of training and competition. It might, therefore, be necessary to study those athletes suffering enforced idleness after meeting some accident such as breaking a leg. It would also be instructive, in endurance athletes, to examine the fibre type composition of muscles that are not directly involved in the training. Top class sprinters tend to have highly developed upper and lower body musculature while it is unusual to see an endurance athlete with highly developed muscles of the upper body, suggesting that somatotype and muscle composition may share a common genetic component.

7.4 Energy reserves and rates of utilization

The central dilemma concerning the selection of fuel for muscular exercise is that there is a choice to be made between the *size* of the reserves and the *rate* at which the energy can be obtained from these stores. In general, the larger the store (i.e. greater endurance) the lower the power output that can be sustained (Table 2) so that in the bath water model (Fig. 7.1) the larger the reservoir the smaller the size of the tap.

The muscle content of ATP, PC and the energy available from glycolysis, is sufficient to sustain activity at a power output equivalent to 80% VO_2max for about 60 seconds. Liver glycogen and glucose in the circulation can sustain this level of effort for about 20 minutes and oxidation of muscle glycogen stores can further sustain the exercise for about one hour. Although there may be massive stores of triglyceride in the body there is a limit to the rate at which this fuel can be utilised. Oxidation of body fat could theoretically support a high level of activity for over 4,000 minutes but in practice nobody can sustain this level for more than a few hours. Untrained subjects can sustain 80% VO$_2$max for only about 30 minutes while a highly motivated trained athlete can sustain this level for the duration of a marathon (about 3 hours). The maximum rate of energy production from the oxidation of fat is about 50% that from the oxidation of carbohydrate. If a subject chooses to exercise at less than 50% VO$_2$max, then the work can be sustained by oxidation of fatty acids for very long periods provided that feet, ankles and knees survive; this is the strategy that "ultradistance" athletes are forced to adopt for their 100-mile and 6-day races.

Energy source	Body store kJ	Time at 80% max (min)	Rate of liberation
Muscle ATP, PC & glycolysis	80	1	1.0
Oxidation of blood glucose	320	4	0.5
Oxidation of liver glycogen	1,500	18	0.5
Oxidation of muscle glycogen	6,000	70	0.5
Oxidation of body fats	33,700	4,018	0.25

Table 7.2 Fuels for exercise. Values are given for the total body stores (kJ), the time the stores would last as the sole source of energy at 80% VO$_2$max, and the relative rates of energy liberation (partly from Newsholme, 1987).

7.5 Strategies for improving performance in endurance exercise

In running a marathon a compromise must be made between the rate at which energy can be liberated and the size of the store being used. From Table 7.2 it can be seen that it is possible to sustain a high power output using muscle glycogen but that reserves are only sufficient for 1 to 1.5 hours exercise. When muscle glycogen is depleted there is no alternative but to oxidise fat which can support power output at only about half that provided by carbohydrates. The time at which the muscle glycogen stores are used up and the body has only fat as a substrate is known as "hitting the wall" and leads to a rapid decline in running speed. In this context there are two ways in which performance in endurance events can be improved.

7.5.1 *Increasing muscle glycogen stores*

One way of improving endurance of exercise at high levels of
oxygen uptake is to increase the muscle glycogen content by the
carbohydrate-loading techniques now commonly used by endurance
runners. Bergstrom and colleagues (1966, 1967) first noted this effect
during an investigation of the rate of glycogen resynthesis after fatiguing
exercise. The subjects exercised one leg to exhaustion while the other
leg acted as a control. It was found that having depleted the test leg of
glycogen, muscle levels were restored after one day. However the
surprising finding was that on the second and third days after exercise
the muscle glycogen was one and half to twice as high as in the control
muscles (Fig. 7.6).

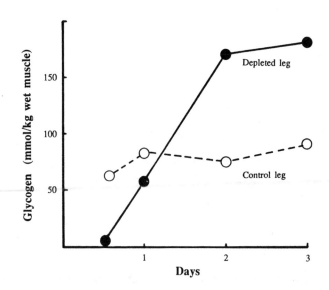

Fig. 7.6 Muscle glycogen following exhaustive exercise. Values are given for the
control and depleted leg, the first biopsy being taken immediately after the exercise
(redrawn from Bergstrom & Hultman, 1966).

Glycogen levels in muscle can be raised by simply feeding a high
carbohydrate diet without any exercise (Fig. 7.7) and there have been
various suggestions that the loading may be enhanced by taking a low
carbohydrate diet for a week before the race followed by a high
carbohydrate diet 24 to 48 hours before the exercise. The optimum
combination of exercise and diet has not been fully evaluated but there
is no doubt that muscle glycogen stores can be significantly elevated
with beneficial effects for running speed and endurance.

7.5.2 *Increased utilization of fats*

The maximum rate of energy production from fat oxidation is such as to limit the power output to 50% VO₂max. If fat oxidation is fully utilised a power output of 80% VO₂max could be achieved if the glycogen stores were to provide the remaining 30%. The limited glycogen store is then used only to "top up" the energy requirement and consequently is used up at about a third of the rate that would be required if glycogen were the only source of energy.

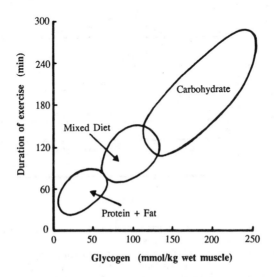

Fig. 7.7 The effect of diet on muscle glycogen and endurance at 75% VO₂max: a low carbohydrate diet containing mainly fat and protein, a mixed diet and a high carbohydrate diet. Note that endurance is related to the muscle glycogen content (redrawn from Bergstrom *et al*, 1967).

If it were possible to utilise fatty acids at a maximum and constant rate from the start of exercise, a high and constant power output could be maintained for a longer time in contrast to the abrupt loss of performance seen if the two fuels are used sequentially (Fig. 7.8).

Fatty acid oxidation is largely controlled by the availability of substrate. In rats a fat meal, followed by an injection of heparin, which raised the plasma free fatty acids, led to a reduction in glycogen utilisation during exercise. The sparing effect of fatty acid oxidation was evident for muscle and liver glycogen and it was found to increase endurance time during running (Rennie *et al*, 1976). Fatty acid oxidation appears to spare carbohydrate by two mechanisms; directly reducing glucose uptake by the tissue and decreasing glycolysis as a consequence of the accumulation of citrate which inhibits phosphofructokinase.

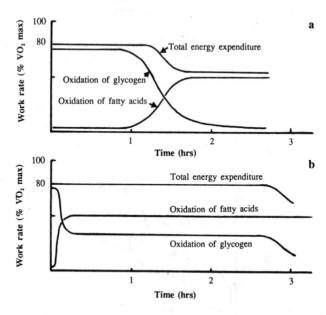

Fig. 7.8   Contribution of fat and carbohydrate oxidation to total energy expenditure during prolonged exercise. **a**, mobilisation of fatty acids late in the exercise means that a workload of 80% VO₂max can only be sustained at the expense of rapid glycogen depletion. **b**, early mobilisation of fatty acids means that glycogen is spared and high power output can be maintained for a longer period.

In normal untrained subjects fatty acids are mobilised and make a significant contribution to the energy requirements only after an hour or so of exercise at a time when glycogen stores are becoming depleted. In contrast, elite endurance athletes have high levels of fat oxidation, with sparing of carbohydrate, during exercise. The utilisation of fat also begins earlier in the exercise. Trained cyclists working at the same percentage VO₂max as untrained subjects were found to have lower plasma lactate and higher plasma free fatty acids than untrained controls indicating a greater use of fats and a shift away from carbohydrate utilisation (Fig. 7.9). The mechanism underlying this adaptation is far from clear. Fat mobilization is largely determined by hormonal changes; catecholamines, cortisol, and growth hormone all activate lipases in adipose tissue. However, measurements of the hormonal responses of trained athletes to exercise tend to show similar or even smaller changes than in untrained subjects. This observation raises the possibility of an adaptation of the catecholamine or other receptors, leading to either an increased density or sensitivity in the target organs of trained subjects.

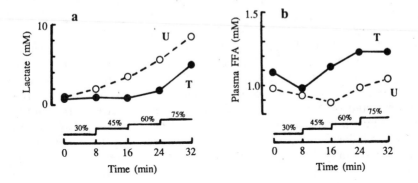

Fig. 7.9 · Metabolic response to exercise in trained (**T**) and untrained (**U**) cyclists undertaking a progressive exercise test. **a**, plasma lactate response is greater in the untrained subjects while, **b**, the trained cyclists mobilised fatty acids earlier in the exercise '(redrawn from Bloom *et al*, 1976).

There is a precedent for hormone receptors to change in sensitivity or number as insulin receptors are known to fluctuate with levels of habitual exercise and diet. Obese, inactive people, especially the elderly, tend to become insulin resistant. The hormones and receptors controlling fatty acid metabolism may be similarly regulated.

Carbohydrate supplements taken before or in the early stages of exercise may be counterproductive in that they will stimulate insulin production and delay the mobilization of fatty acids, although in the latter stages of a marathon they may confer some benefit in maintaining blood glucose when liver glycogen is depleted. Caffeine, in the form of strong coffee, can stimulate lipolysis and probably helps to mobilise fatty acids early in the exercise.

7.6 Cardiovascular or peripheral limitations to exercise

There is some doubt as to what is the limiting factor for maximum aerobic exercise. The two broad possibilities are either that the heart can only circulate a limiting volume of oxygenated blood to the working muscles, or, alternatively, the pump is working within its capabilities but the muscle itself is limited in the amount of oxygen that it can extract and utilise. Using a modified cycle ergometer with only one pedal it is possible to measure the oxygen cost of maximum one-legged exercise and to compare this with conventional two-legged exercise. If the limitation was peripheral, i.e. in the ability of muscle to extract oxygen, then doubling the amount of working muscle ought to double the oxygen uptake. Conversely if the central pump was limiting then increasing the muscle bulk would not be expected to increase the oxygen used. It is generally found that VO_2max measured with two legs is less than twice the VO_2max obtained when exercising only one leg, the implication being that the central pump supplying blood is not sufficient to supply the maximum requirements of two working legs. The precise proportion of maximum that can be achieved with one leg exercise varies with the cardiac output and the size of the legs; for a heavily muscled weightlifter with a relatively small cardiac output, VO_2max may be achieved with exercise of only one leg, while an endurance athlete with small leg muscles and a large heart may be able to double the one legged VO_2max by using two legs.

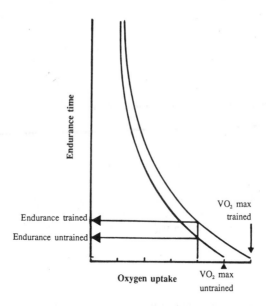

Fig. 7.10   Endurance times at different workloads. Training has a relatively small percentage effect on VO_2max but makes a large difference to the endurance at submaximal levels of exercise.

It is a well known that VO_2max obtained by leg exercise cannot be improved by including work with the arms. It is estimated that for a subject of average stature, activation of about 30% of the body musculature is sufficient to reach the limit of the central pump and achieve whole body VO_2max. The implication of this observation is that skeletal muscle is over provided with capillaries and mitochondrial enzymes; nevertheless an increase in these is one of the features seen after endurance training. The answer to this paradox may be the observation that endurance training has a far greater effect on endurance at submaximum levels of exercise than it does on VO_2max (Fig. 7.10).

Training might increase VO_2max by 30% at most yet endurance at submaximal work loads may increase three to fourfold. This is because the relationship between the level of activity and endurance is hyperbolic (Fig. 7.10) so that small changes in the intercept on the y axis will have a large effect for submaximal endurance. The substrate used by the muscles will have a major effect on the shape of the curve, the more fatty acid that can be utilised, the steeper will be the relationship. The increase in capillary density and mitochondrial enzymes may be a way of increasing fatty acid utilization during submaximal exercise.

7.7 Temperature regulation and dehydration

Temperature regulation and dehydration are two factors that affect performance in endurance events, especially in warm conditions. Elevated core temperature severely reduces endurance. High temperatures increase the rate of energy expenditure in the muscle for a given workload, making it less efficient, and may also divert blood away from the working muscles to the skin. The decrease in performance in hot conditions can be very marked and it is not established that the metabolic changes are sufficient to account fully for the decrease in performance. This raises the possibility of a central response to increased core temperature. Training results in an adaptation of temperature regulation, sweating beginning earlier and being more copious in the trained subject. Although trained subjects may be better able to dissipate heat, they are no more tolerant of actual increases in core temperature.

Dehydration *per se* will reduce performance by lowering the maximum heart rate, but the main effect is to limit the rate of sweat production and impair evaporative heat loss. Loss of body fluid or increased plasma osmolarity reduce sweating and inhibit vasodilation. These effects are appreciable after a loss of fluid equal to 1% of body weight. Losses of 5% body weight are not uncommon during marathons in warm conditions and clearly it is important to minimise the loss of body fluids. To do this the athlete should be fully hydrated before the race, drinking a large quantity of water about two hours before the start and then taking frequent small drinks during the race. Thirst is not a good indicator of dehydration and consequently drinks should be taken at regular intervals irrespective of feelings of thirst. Cold water appears to be the best drink; electrolyte supplements are not necessary during a marathon and can be detrimental if they increase the osmolarity of the plasma. Carbohydrate supplements may cause water loss by drawing water into the intestine by osmosis.

7.8 References and further reading

Åstrand, P.-O., Engström, L., Eriksson, B.O., Karlberg, P., Nylander, I., Saltin, B. & Thorén, C. (1963). Girl swimmers. *Acta Paediatrica* (Suppl **147**).

Bergström, J., Hermansen, L., Hultman, E. & Saltin, B. (1967). Diet, muscle glycogen and physical performance. *Acta Physiologica Scandinavia* **71**, 140-50.

Bergström, J. & Hultman, E. (1966). Muscle glycogen synthesis after exercise: an enhancing factor localized to muscle cells in man. *Nature* **210**, 309-10.

Bloom, S.R., Johnson, R.H., Park, D.M., Rennie, M.J. & Sulaiman, W.R. (1976). Differences in the metabolic and hormonal response to exercise between racing cyclists and untrained individuals. *Journal of Physiology* **258**, 1-18.

Ekblom, B. (1969). Effect of physical training on oxygen transport system in man. *Acta Physiologica Scandinavia* (Suppl **328**).

Galbo, H. (1983). *Hormonal and Metabolic Adaptation to Exercise*, Stuttgart & New York, Georg Thieme Verlag.

Harrison, M.H. (1987). Fluid balance as a limiting factor for exercise. In: *Exercise: Benefits, Limits and Adaptations*, ed. D. Macleod *et al*. London, E. & F.N. Spon Ltd, pp. 367-87.

Hudlicka, O. (1988). Capillary growth: role of mechanical factors. *News in Physiological Sciences* **3**, 117-20.

Newsholme, E.A. (1987). Application of metabolic logic to the questions of causes of fatigue in marathon races. In: *Exercise: Benefits, Limits and Adaptations*, ed. D. Macleod *et al*. London, E. & F.N. Spon Ltd, pp. 181-198.

Rennie, M.J., Winder, W.W. & Holloszy, O. (1976). A sparing effect of increased plasma fatty acids on muscle and liver glycogen content in the exercising rat. *Biochemical Journal* **156**, 647-55.

Saltin, B. & Gollnick, P.D. (1983). Skeletal muscle adaptability: significance for metabolism and performance. In: *Handbook of Physiology, Section 10, Skeletal muscle*. ed. L.D. Peachey, R.H. Adrian & S.R. Geiger, Bethesda, American Physiological Society, pp. 555-631.

Savard, G., Kiens, B. & Saltin, B. (1987). Central cardiovascular factors as limits to endurnace; with a note on the distinction between maximal oxygen uptake and endurance fitness. In: *Exercise: Benefits, Limits and Adaptations*, ed. D. Macleod *et al*. London, E. & F.N. Spon Ltd, pp. 162-77.

Thomson, M., Stone, A., Ginsburg, A.D. & Hamilton, P. (1982). O_2 transport during exercise following blood reinfusion. *Journal of Applied Physiology* **53**, 1213-19.

Wasserman, D.H. & Vranic, M. (1986). Interactions between insulin, glucagon and catecholamines in the regulation of glucose production and uptake during exercise: physiology and diabetes. In: *Biochemistry of Exercise VI,* ed. B. Saltin. International Series on Sports Sciences, Vol 16. Champaign, Ill., Human Kinetics Publishers. pp. 167-79.

Chapter 8

FATIGUE

There are two types of question generally asked about fatigue. The first concerns the site of failure: does the loss of performance arise because of a malfunction in, for instance, the neural pathways, at the neuromuscular junction or in any of the various processes concerned with the generation of force within the muscle fibre? The second category of question is about the nature of the change that leads to the failure. If the failure is of central processes, is it caused by pain or low blood sugar? If within the muscle fibre, is it due to a low concentration of ATP, high phosphate, H^+ or other metabolite?

8.1 The definition of fatigue

The first problem we encounter when discussing fatigue is that the word itself has a number of different meanings tired, exhausted, over-used, disinclined, etc. Most of these words describe sensations which occur as a consequence of muscular activity of one sort or another but it is also possible to experience fatigue without prolonged activity. It can be more tiring to walk slowly round an over-heated and crowded exhibition than to walk briskly up a hill on a fine day, yet the amount of work done and energy dissipated will be far greater in the latter activity. It is important, therefore, when considering fatigue to be clear about which particular aspect is under discussion.

Muscular fatigue is a loss of the ability to generate force, but such a simple definition is complicated by the fact that the extent of fatigue may vary according to the method of testing. The extent of fatigue may appear greater for voluntary contractions than for tetanic stimulation, or may differ according to whether the muscle is tested at one frequency of stimulation compared to another, or if the muscle is allowed to shorten rather than being held isometric. To add to the confusion, if a fatigued muscle is stretched it may be able to sustain *more* force than a fresh muscle. It is important, therefore, in each situation to specify the type of change in muscle function that is being described as "fatigue".

Most experimental work has been based on the measurement of isometric contractions and in the first part of this chapter we will consider changes in isometric force during contractions lasting for about

60 seconds. Later sections will examine how these changes may affect the behaviour of muscles during other forms of exercise.

8.2 Central factors

To sustain a maximum isometric contraction requires considerable concentration and effort. After about 10s, feelings of discomfort develop and by 30-45s the burning becomes so intense that the subject has little idea how much force the muscle is generating. It is essential, therefore, in this type of experiment to have some form of visual feedback to give the subject a target at which to aim. In the absence of visual feedback, where the subject has to rely on sensory information alone, force rapidly declines.

8.2.1 *The sense of effort*
The origins of the sense of muscular effort are poorly understood. There are basically two schools of thought on the subject. One opinion is that signals originating in the motor centre radiate to the centre responsible for the perception of effort (Fig. 8.1a). The alternative point of view is that afferents from sensory receptors in the muscle give information about muscle activity in much the same way as our knowledge of limb position comes from receptors signalling joint angle (Fig. 8.1b).

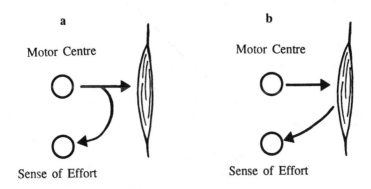

Fig. 8.1 Possible origins of the sense of muscular effort. **a**, sense of effort due to a collateral pathway reaching a conscious centre. **b**, sense of effort due to afferent information from the active muscle.

In the one case, therefore, our sense of effort is derived from what the higher centres are *telling* the muscle to do, in the other it comes from what the muscle is *actually* doing. In either case there is considerable scope for modification of the perception of effort by afferent information coming from the cardiovascular and respiratory systems, or from joints and skin. Other factors such as core temperature and the elusive quality of central drive or motivation all affect our perception and response to the sensations associated with muscular exercise.

8.2.2 *Central factors during fatigue*

All voluntary contractions involve activity of the central nervous system and it is quite likely that this central nervous activity is modified during the course of sustained activity, either because of short-term adaptations within the central nervous system or as a reflex response to changes in afferent input.

Failure of central mechanisms can be assessed by superimposing electrical stimulation on voluntary contractions. Stimulation at various points along the chain of command (Fig. 8.2) checks the integrity of the chain distal to the point of stimulation.

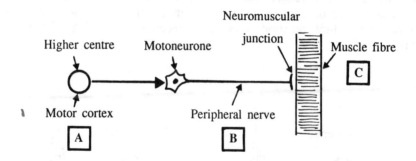

Fig. 8.2 The chain of command linking the higher centres with muscular contraction. The letters **A**, **B** & **C** refer to the sites where electrical stimulation can be used to test the function of the chain.

The motor cortex can be stimulated directly using high voltages and electrodes on the scalp or high magnetic fields generated by discharging large capacitors through a coil (Fig. 8.2, **A**). By carefully placing the electrodes over certain areas of the motor cortex, specific muscles, or groups of muscles, can be activated. A similar technique can be used to stimulate motoneurones in the spinal cord. These methods are rather specialised and require care in using the high voltages. The information gained is largely limited to recording the force and electrical signal of single twitches and its main use is in the investigation of neurological disorders to establish whether there is a functional connection between central nervous system and muscle.

A more widely applicable technique is to stimulate the peripheral motor nerves (**B** in Fig. 8.2). This can be achieved with a small button electrode placed over the appropriate nerve, such as the femoral nerve supplying the quadriceps or the ulnar or median nerves supplying muscles of the hand. An alternative is to activate the nerves through the skin (percutaneous stimulation). Large moistened pad electrodes are placed on the skin to stimulate the peripheral branches of the motor nerve as they enter the muscle.

Stimulating the anatomical nerve has the advantage that the whole muscle can be activated, whereas with percutaneous stimulation it is usually only possible to stimulate a portion of the muscle. In the latter case the assumption has to be made that the portion stimulated is representative of the of the whole, that is, the muscle is functionally homogeneous.

If the muscle is stimulated with single pulses during a voluntary contraction the size of the superimposed twitch will be inversely proportional to the degree to which the muscle is activated (see Chapter 6, Fig. 6.6), and this technique can be used to test the extent of central activation during a fatiguing contraction. However the twitch itself can change in size and shape and it may be more appropriate to use tetanic stimulation (Fig. 8.3).

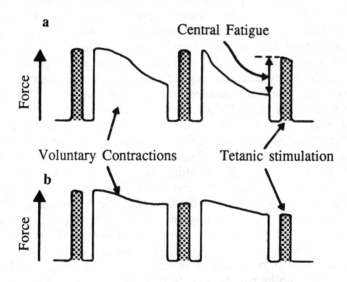

Fig. 8.3 Voluntary contractions with interposed tetanic stimulation. **a**, fatigue partly due to central failure: note the greater fall in voluntary force compared to tetanic force. **b**, voluntary and tetanic force decline in parallel showing no central fatigue.

After about 30-45s of a maximum isometric contraction, pain makes it difficult to concentrate and maintain full activation. For sustained maximum voluntary contractions of the quadriceps, central fatigue has been shown to be a factor leading to loss of force in many subjects towards the end of a 60s contraction (Bigland-Ritchie *et al*, 1978), but with similar contractions of the adductor pollicis of the hand there is little or no evidence of central failure. This type of fatigue has only been examined during relatively simple forms of exercise involving one muscle group. It is not known if it is possible to fully activate several muscle groups as they fatigue, especially if they are involved in a complex series of movements.

8.3 The neuromuscular junction

The idea that the neuromuscular junction may fail during fatigue is attractive since exhausting the stores of neurotransmitter provides an obvious mechanism. At the start of a train of impulses the number of acetylcholine quanta released into the synaptic cleft falls but then comes to an equilibrium depending on the frequency of release (i.e. the rate of stimulation) and the rate at which acetyl choline is resynthesised and made available for release. Where, as a result of poisoning (e.g. with curare or hemicholium) or disease (e.g. myasthenia gravis), the number of quanta released is reduced or the postsynaptic membrane is of a reduced sensitivity, the fresh muscle may be close to the threshold for successful transmission. The first response to a train of impulses could be quite normal but, as the transmitter release decreases, the quantity may fall below the threshold required to evoke an action potential in the post-synaptic membrane and, consequently, force will decline.

Working with an isolated rat phrenic nerve and diaphragm preparation, Krnjvick & Miledi (1958) concluded that at frequencies of around 10Hz there was little likelihood of any failure, but that with higher frequencies breakdown might occur either as a result of a failure of conduction along the fine branches of the motor axons or from a failure of the end plate potential to propagate along the surface membrane of the fibre. To test NMJ function it is necessary to stimulate the muscle fibres directly, bypassing the neuromuscular junction (C in Fig. 8.2). By comparing the result of stimulating through the nerve to the force generated by direct stimulation of the muscle fibres, an estimate can be made of the extent of neuromuscular junction failure. This procedure can be used with isolated animal muscle preparations but it is difficult with human muscles *in situ*. Percutaneous stimulation with acceptable voltages activates the muscle only through the nerve endings, and to activate the muscle fibres directly requires very high voltages which, as with direct stimulation of the motor cortex, poses obvious difficulties.

The effectiveness of electrical propagation across the neuromuscular junction in human subjects can be assessed more easily by stimulating the motor nerve and recording the muscle action potential. This signal is known as the *M wave* and is the summation of individual fibre action potentials in the part of the muscle near the electrode. Neuromuscular junction failure in a number of fibres will reduce the amplitude of the M wave. Merton (1954) was the first to use this technique to study fatigue in normal subjects and found that while the force progressively declined during a sustained voluntary contraction, the muscle action potential remained constant, thus demonstrating the integrity of neuromuscular transmission. This conclusion was disputed by Stephens and Taylor (1972) who presented conflicting evidence. Since then Bigland-Ritchie and colleagues (1982) have systematically examined the question of NMJ failure and have been unable to find any evidence of failure during maximal isometric contractions of up to 60s.

8.4 Peripheral factors

Fatiguing exercise entails large metabolic fluxes and changes in the concentration of muscle metabolites. It is understandable, therefore, that a good deal of work in the last thirty years has been directed to finding an explanation for fatigue in terms of altered metabolite levels affecting force production by actin and myosin.

For an investigation of force and metabolite changes the first problem is to find a reliable method for measuring labile muscle metabolites.

For chemical methods the tissue is frozen, extracted, usually with acid, and metabolites measured in the neutralised extract. Analytical methods such as linked enzyme assays can be made very sensitive and, with refinement, it is possible to make measurements on fragments of single fibres. Using a biopsy needle, human muscle working *in vivo* can be sampled and the needle plus sample of muscle rapidly plunged into isopentane, or similar refrigerant, cooled with liquid nitrogen. Two or three samples can be taken from one muscle (usually the quadriceps) during the course on an experiment. At best, the time between taking the sample and freezing is around 5 seconds, an appreciable interval for metabolite changes to take place. Isolated muscle preparations can be frozen more rapidly, usually by flattening the muscle between two metal blocks cooled in liquid nitrogen. Obviously, using this method, only one measurement can be made on each muscle.

Nuclear Magnetic Resonance spectroscopy (NMR) is increasingly used to measure phosphorus metabolites in muscle. In this technique phosphorus nuclei are caused to process in a magnetic field and in so doing they radiate energy at radio frequencies. The frequency of the radiation is characteristic of the chemical compound of which it is a part and the amplitude of the signal is proportional to the quantity of the compound. Thus a Fourier analysis of the signal, which gives the energy at different frequencies, yields information about the composition and concentration of phosphorus metabolites present in the tissue. Developments in the technology of large superconducting magnets have led to the manufacture of NMR machines into which small animals, babies or adult arms and legs can be inserted. The largest magnets can accommodate a whole body but these instruments are used primarily for medical imaging. The great advantage of NMR is that measurements are non-invasive, and since there is no damage to the tissue the measurements can be repeated (Fig. 8.4).

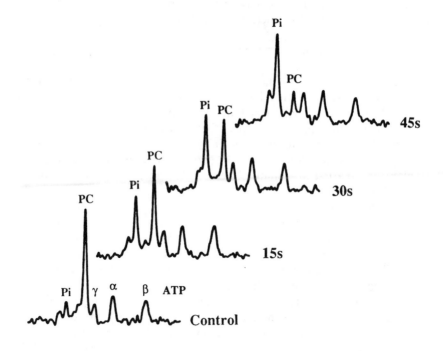

Fig. 8.4 NMR spectroscopy used to measure phosphorus metabolites in human muscle (first dorsal interosseous). Averaged spectra from a fully rested muscle (Control) and from a muscle after 15, 30 and 45s of maximum voluntary contraction. Note the progressive decrease in phosphocreatine (PC) and increase in inorganic phosphate (Pi) peaks. The α, β and γ peaks of ATP remain constant.

The main disadvantage of NMR is that the radio signal is very weak and a number of spectra have to be averaged to obtain reliable data, for example, a minimum of one minute is required to obtain acceptable measurements from human hand or leg muscles. Consequently rapid changes in metabolites cannot be followed.

The internal pH of the muscle fibre can be estimated from the position of the Pi peak in the NMR spectra. As pH changes so the charge on Pi varies and the characteristic frequency will alter. Lactate cannot be directly measured from the phosphorus spectrum but, assuming the pH change to be solely the result of glycolysis, the change in lactate can be calculated from the pH shift by making reasonable assumptions about the nature and quantity of intracellular buffers. The main buffers are protein-bound histidine, carnosine, bicarbonate and, in fatigued muscle, Pi.

An alternative technique for investigating the relationship between metabolite concentrations and force production is to use skinned preparations, either single fibres or small bundles. The composition of the external incubation medium can be altered and the effect on force observed. Single fibres can be mechanically skinned by removing the surface membrane with a needle, but the more common method is chemical skinning, using a detergent which makes the surface membrane permeable. Dissecting and handling single fibres from amphibian muscle is difficult and it is very difficult with mammalian muscle where there is more connective tissue. For mammalian preparations, small bundles of fibres, often from the psoas muscle, are commonly used. Another technical problem is to maintain constant concentrations of metabolites throughout the preparation. ATP will be used up during a contraction and fresh ATP has to diffuse from the bulk of the medium into the centre of the fibre while ADP and Pi have to diffuse out. To avoid depleting ATP in this way, high concentrations of PC and creatine kinase are included in the bathing medium but, as hydrolysis of ATP and PC proceeds, Pi will accumulate in the centre of the preparation.

The changes in muscle metabolites during a sustained maximal isometric contraction are shown for an isolated mouse soleus muscle (Fig. 8.5) and the human first dorsal interosseous, studied *in situ* (Fig. 8.6). For the mouse, muscle metabolites were measured by chemical methods and for the human muscle by NMR. The change in force during the exercise can also be seen. Despite the differences in species and analytical methods the results for the two preparations are basically similar. Phosphocreatine falls rapidly during the first 15s and there is a concomitant rise in inorganic phosphate (Pi). Lactate increases in a linear fashion throughout the contraction. The lactate was measured directly in the mouse muscles but would have to be calculated from the pH measurements in the human muscles.

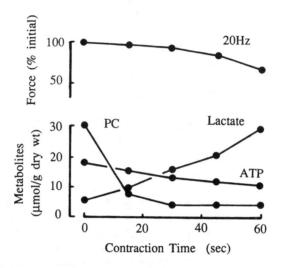

Fig. 8.5   Muscle metabolites during a sustained contraction. Isolated mouse soleus muscle (25°C) poisoned with cyanide and stimulated at 20Hz (Edwards *et al*, 1975).

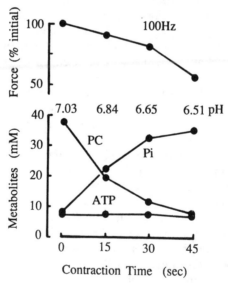

Fig. 8.6   Muscle metabolites during a sustained contraction. Human first dorsal interosseous, maximum voluntary contractions for 15s and tested by stimulating at 100Hz. NMR spectra collected over the next 3 minutes (Fig 8.4). The cycle was repeated three times with the muscle ischaemic throughout. Numbers above the metabolite values are the intracellular pH (Cady *et al*, 1989a).

The fact that glycolysis appears to be activated from the start of the contraction is noteworthy as there are suggestions in the literature of a delay, the so-called "alactacid" phase. In both preparations it is possible to measure the ATP directly and it is clear (as has been shown in many other studies) that, for contractions of normal muscle lasting about a minute, there is no major alteration in content.

The nature and extent of the metabolite changes illustrated here are typical of results for a variety of preparations obtained with different analytical methods. We must now consider the significance of these changes for force production.

8.4.1 *Metabolite changes and force production*

8.4.1.1 *Adenosine triphosphate* ATP is intimately involved in cross-bridge function with the binding of ATP to myosin causing dissociation of the actomyosin complex (Chapter 2, Section 2.5). In the absence of ATP, cross-bridges remain in the attached state which is the reason for the muscle stiffness after death (*rigor mortis*). Fatigued muscle relaxes slowly and in some circumstances resting tension will rise, and it is natural to wonder whether this signifies a low ATP and the onset of rigor. Measurements of ATP levels in fatigued muscle, as in Figs. 8.5 and 8.6, show, at most, only small reductions in ATP content, while experiments with skinned preparations demonstrate that force generation is virtually independent of ATP in the range of concentrations that would be expected in normal and fatigued muscle (Fig. 8.7). Force loss, therefore, is unlikely to be a consequence of low ATP as a substrate affecting the cross-bridge cycle.

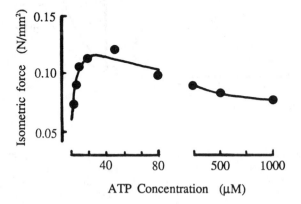

Fig. 8.7 Isometric tension as a function of ATP concentration in skinned rabbit psoas muscle bundles (redrawn from Cooke & Bialek, 1979).

The free energy that can be obtained by hydrolysis of ATP (affinity) will depend on the relative concentrations of the various reaction products, ADP, Pi and H^+. It is possible that even if there is only a small change in ATP during fatigue, the affinity could decrease significantly and, with it, the amount of force generated.   Dawson *et al* (1978) calculated the change in affinity during a fatiguing contraction and found it did not correlate well with change in force.   They did, however, conclude that it was related to the slowing of the rate of relaxation (see below).

8.4.1.2 *Intracellular pH* A decrease of intracellular pH as a result of glycolysis and H^+ accumulation can have a number of effects. High H^+ concentrations in skinned preparations lead to a reduction in the maximum force generated at saturating Ca^{2+} concentrations, affecting, in some way, the attachment of myosin and actin or a stage in the cross bridge-cycle. At pH 6.5, about the lowest value found in normally fatigued muscle, the reduction in maximum force is around 10 to 30%, with fast muscle being more affected than slow (Fig. 8.8; Donaldson & Hermansen, 1978; Fabiato & Fabiato, 1978).

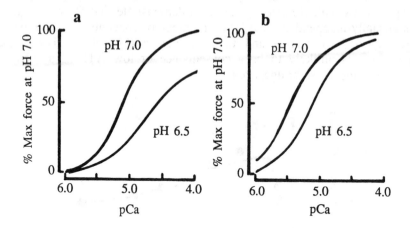

Fig. 8.8 The effect of pH on force production in skinned muscle bundles. Forces at different calcium concentrations (pCa) are given relative to the maximum force at pH 7.0. **a**, fast adductor magnus bundles. **b**, slow soleus muscle fibres. Results obtained in the presence of 1mM Mg^{2+} (redrawn from Donaldson & Hermansen, 1978).

Another action of H^+ in skinned cardiac and skeletal muscle preparations is that low pH deceases the sensitivity of troponin for Ca^{2+}, shifting the pCa/force curve to the right (Fig. 8.8). During maximal activation this may be of little consequence as there seems to be an excess of calcium released from the SR at high frequencies of stimulation. However the reduced sensitivity to Ca^{2+} could lead to a lower force during partial activation either because of low stimulation frequencies or disruption of the EC coupling mechanism.

H^+ may have an indirect action by inhibiting glycolysis at the level of phosphofructokinase which will reduce the production of ATP. Although it has been argued here (Section 8.4.1.1) that changes in ATP have little effect on force generation by the contractile proteins, there are other processes concerned with ion transport and membrane excitability that are ATP dependent and could influence the force generated by an intact muscle.

Finally H^+ may have an effect on the cross-bridge, either directly, or by changing the charge on Pi, this possibility is discussed below (Section 8.4.1.3).

While a *fall* in pH may play some part in the development of fatigue it cannot be the only cause. Fatigue develops even more rapidly than normal when glycolysis is absent and no rise in hydrogen ion occurs, as in muscle poisoned by iodoacetate or in patients with myophosphorylase deficiency. In these muscles pH *rises* slightly during the contraction as the result of PC hydrolysis and liberation of Pi which is a significant source of buffering capacity in the active muscle (Cady *et al*, 1989).

8.4.1.3 *Phosphate* Inorganic phosphate accumulates in fatigued muscle and, as a reaction product of the actomyosin ATPase, might be expected to affect cross-bridge cycling.

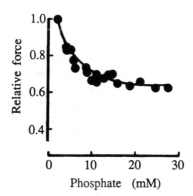

Fig. 8.9 Isometric force of skinned single fibres as a function of Pi in the bathing medium (redrawn from Cooke & Pate, 1985).

In skinned cardiac and skeletal muscle preparations phosphate has been shown to have a marked effect on force generation (Cooke & Pate, 1985; Kentish, 1986), with most of the effect being seen with an increase of phosphate from low levels to about 10mM (Fig. 8.9).

With intact skeletal muscle, however, an increase of 10mM Pi occurs within the first 15s of contraction, during which time there is comparatively little fall in isometric force (Fig. 8.5 & 8.6). Force begins to fall rapidly from about 30 to 45s, at a time when total phosphate is changing very little, but pH is decreasing.

The pK of the reaction $HPO_4^{2-} + H^+ \rightleftharpoons H_2PO_4^-$ is close to 7 so that the proportions of the mono and dibasic forms of phosphate will vary greatly with change of pH in the physiological range. At rest with an intracellular pH of just over 7, approximately two-thirds of the phosphate is in the dibasic form but as the muscle fatigues, and pH falls, the proportion will change so that by pH 6.5 approximately two-thirds will be in the monobasic form. The appearance of monobasic phosphate in the fibre will therefore lag behind that of the total phosphate and correlate more closely with the change in force. With skinned preparations a relationship between monobasic phosphate and isometric force has been described; 20 mM, which is near to the maximum concentration found in a fatigued muscle (Fig. 8.6), being sufficient to reduce the force by about 50% (Nosek *et al*, 1987). In normal muscle the monobasic phosphate can rise to about 25mM but where glycolysis is absent or is poisoned and there is no change in pH, the monobasic phosphate will rise to only about 12mM. Where glycolysis is absent, loss of force is as great, if not greater, than for normal muscle (Cady *et al*, 1989a). A combination of increased phosphate and decreased pH almost certainly has some effect on force generation, but the extent to which it can explain fatigue remains to be resolved.

8.4.2 *Slowing of relaxation*

Slowing of relaxation from an isometric contraction is characteristic of acutely fatigued muscle. The half-time of the exponential phase typically increases two to threefold as a result of fatiguing voluntary contractions (Fig. 8.10), and similar changes occur as a result of stimulated contractions in isolated muscle preparations. The relaxation phase is electrically silent and is not the type of slow relaxation seen with myotonia where the muscle fibre membrane fires repetitively. Under anaerobic conditions there is little or no recovery from this slowing. When circulation is restored to ischaemic human muscle, recovery has a half time of about 60s, which is similar to the time course of phosphocreatine resynthesis although an effect of pH, which remains low during the first one to two minutes of recovery, can be demonstrated (Cady *et al*, 1989b).

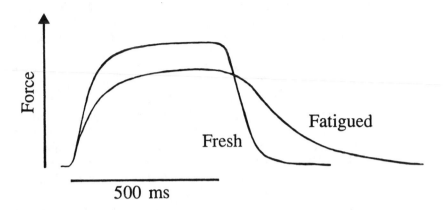

Fig. 8.10 Relaxation of force at the end of a brief tetanus of fresh muscle and after 30s fatiguing contraction. Human first dorsal interosseous of the hand (Cady *et al*, 1989b).

Contractile slowing leads to a reduction in tetanic fusion frequency with a shift to the left of the force-frequency relationship (Fig. 8.11). Muscles are seldom excited at their maximum tetanic frequencies so that in most types of exercise they are working on the steep portion of the curve. In these circumstances a slowing of relaxation allows the same force to be generated at a lower frequency of stimulation.

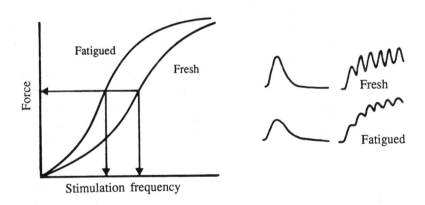

Fig. 8.11 The effect of slow relaxation in fatigued muscle on the force/frequency relationship. The insert shows the effect of fatigue on the degree of fusion; on the left, single twitches; on the right, stimulation at 7Hz.

The mechanism causing the slowing is not known but there are two main possibilities. The first is that the slowing is due to a reduced rate of cross-bridge detachment. This implies a change in the cross-bridge which should be reflected in the force velocity curve of fatigued muscle. There is evidence, in animal muscle studies, of a decrease in the maximum velocity of shortening with the onset of fatigue at a time when relaxation is also changing (Crow & Kushmerick, 1984; de Haan *et al*, 1989; Section 8.6.2.1). A reduction in ATP or an increase in ADP would both decrease shortening velocity by reducing the rate of detachment of the cross-bridge at the end of the power stroke. However, the concentrations at which these changes are seen (less than 1 mM ATP or about 4mM ADP) are outside the normal physiological range. It is most unlikely that in fatigued normal muscle ATP would ever fall below about 4-3mM or ADP rise above 0.5mM.

The second mechanism concerns calcium reaccumulation by the sarcoplasmic reticulum, an ATP-dependent process which could be slowed in adverse metabolic circumstances. Dawson *et al* (1978) found that changes in relaxation correlated with change in the affinity of ATP splitting and suggested that calcium pumping may be critically dependent on the free energy available from ATP.

Although the simple exponential form of relaxation suggests a single underlying biochemical process, evidence is accumulating that there are two processes that can cause slowing. Decreased pH due to H^+ accumulation probably slows the cross-bridge cycle while changes in phosphorus metabolites lead to a slow reaccumulation of calcium by the sarcolpasmic reticulum (Cady *et al*, 1989b).

Since the 1960s there has been continued interest in the relationship between muscle metabolite levels and the generation of force but results have always been tantalising, with so many possibilities but no particular change that could be uniquely identified as the cause of fatigue. There is no doubt that metabolic changes do influence force production as a poisoned or anoxic muscle fails rapidly, yet the chemical changes that are measured are probably not sufficient to cause a change in the function of the actin and myosin. Consequently interest has turned to other steps in the chain of events leading to force generation in the intact muscle fibre.

8.4.3 *Electrical activity in the muscle membrane*

During a prolonged tetanus the time course of force loss depends, in part, on the frequency of stimulation. At high frequencies (80-100Hz in human muscles), force is maintained for only a few seconds before declining to 10 to 20% of its initial value by about 30 seconds. In contrast, when a muscle is stimulated at 20Hz the force remains almost constant for 60s or longer (Fig. 8.12a). After about 15s more force can be produced by stimulating the muscle at 20Hz even though this frequency produced only 60 to 70% of the maximum force in the fresh muscle.

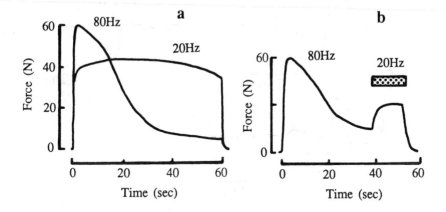

Fig. 8.12 Force loss at two frequencies of stimulation in human adductor pollicis. **a**, muscle stimulated continuously at 20 or 80Hz. **b**, muscle stimulated at 80Hz initially and the frequency then reduced to 20Hz.

At a time when there is considerable force loss as a result of stimulation at high frequency, reducing the stimulation frequency leads to a rapid increase in force (Fig. 8.12b). The force recovers more rapidly than metabolite resynthesis is likely to occur. Very similar behaviour is seen when isolated, curarized muscle preparations are stimulated directly, indicating that the failure is a feature of the muscle membranes and not the neuromuscular junction (Jones *et al*, 1979). This failure is associated with a slowing, and ultimately failure, of the muscle action potential (Bigland-Ritchie *et al*, 1979; Fig. 8.13a).

It is possible that changes in the muscle cation concentration occur during high frequency stimulation, causing a loss of membrane excitability leading to a reduced force. There are large potassium fluxes from working muscle and extracellular concentrations can be as high as 8 to 9mM (Hnik *et al*, 1976; Sjogaard *et al*, 1985). The potassium concentration within the depths of the T tubules must be considerably higher since this is where the majority of K is released and diffusion along the narrow tubules is restricted.

Increasing the potassium ion concentration in the extracelluar medium of an isolated muscle causes a rapid loss of force and slowing of the action potential conduction velocity (Fig. 8.13b), mimicking those seen in fatigue of human muscle.

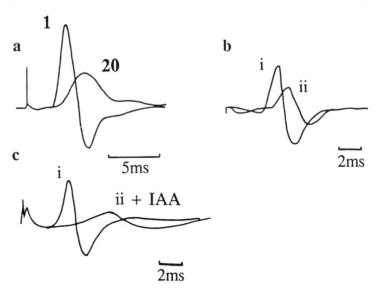

Fig. 8.13   Changes in the action potential waveform. **a,** human adductor pollicis, action potentials recorded after 1 and 20s stimulation at 50Hz. **b,** isolated mouse diaphragm, i. action potential of fresh muscle in medium containing 4mM K⁺ and ii. medium containing 15mM K⁺. **c,** mouse diaphragm preparation, i. action potential from fresh muscle, ii. 3 minutes after poisoning with iodoacetic acid (IAA).

These observations suggest that the muscle fibre membrane becomes depolarised during high-frequency stimulation (Jones & Bigland-Ritchie, 1986), which direct measurements of membrane potential in single fibres confirm, the potential falling from -80mV to -40mV in about 10s when stimulated at 70Hz (Lannergren & Westerblad, 1986, 1987).   In a working muscle there are two factors that could contribute to a fall in membrane potential.   One is the accumulation of K^+ in the extracelluar space (and a smaller proportional reduction in intracellular K^+).   The second possible cause is a metabolic change which could directly affect membrane characteristics and also influence the rate at which the membrane Na^+,K^+ transport mechanism acts to redress the ionic imbalance.   The fact that similar slowing and failure of the action potential can be seen in muscle that is poisoned with iodoacetate (Fig. 8.13c) suggests that this mechanism may be playing a role in fatigue.

High-frequency stimulation is not a natural occurrence in everyday life (see below), which raises the question as to whether membrane depolarization is a feature of normal fatiguing contractions.   Certainly the drastic changes seen in surface-recorded action potentials as a result of high-frequency stimulation are not seen during voluntary contractions. There is, however, some slowing of the action potential wave form which could arise from electrical changes in the T tubular membranes, but it is not possible with present techniques to measure changes in the T tubules, as opposed to the surface membrane. The likelihood is that K^+ accumulation will be highest in the interior of the fibre, where diffusion distances are greatest, and that during high-force contractions the central portion of the T tubular network may become inexcitable. This change will result in a fibre where the central myofibrils are no longer activated and producing force.

8.5 Motor unit firing frequency

During a maximum voluntary contraction (MVC) of the adductor pollicis individual motoneurones discharge at different rates, generally ranging from about 10 to 50Hz, and it has been shown that the mean frequency declines during fatiguing contractions. This decline is accompanied by a slowing of the muscle relaxation rate, which lowers the tetanic fusion frequency (Fig. 8.14).

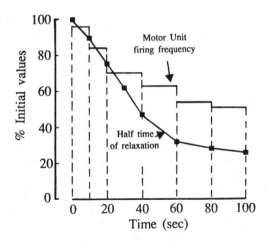

Fig. 8.14 Changes in mean motor unit firing rates recorded from fine wire electrodes in the muscle compared with changes in relaxation rate during a fatiguing maximum voluntary contraction of human muscle. Values are expressed as a percentage of the values in fresh muscle.

The slow relaxation has the effect of maintaining isometric force despite the reduced rate of motoneurone firing (Fig. 8.11).

These observations suggest that for a fatigued muscle the motoneurone firing rates during a maximum voluntary contraction may be regulated to match changes in muscle contractile speed. A possible advantage of this change in firing frequency is that it would avoid the problems associated with high frequency stimulation, described above, where K^+ builds up in the extracellular spaces, reducing the excitability of the muscle. If the muscle is kept ischaemic there is no metabolic recovery and the motoneurone firing frequency remains low and the relaxation slow. There may be a reflex mechanism slowing motor unit firing in response to some change in the fatigued muscle (Bigland-Ritchie *et al*, 1986), and there are many receptors that might signal changes in a fatigued muscle. Group III and group IV free nerve endings (see Chapter 10, Table 10.1) respond vigorously to many of the metabolites which accumulate and possibly to changes in the contractile properties of muscles. These nerve endings are implicated in cardiovascular responses to exercise and have powerful inputs to inhibitory motoneurones. In addition they reduce the discharge rates of γ-motoneurones and therefore seem ideally suited to mediate a reflex which modulates motoneurone firing rates during fatigue.

8.6 Fatigue during dynamic or prolonged exercise

In the first part of this chapter we have concentrated on the loss of force during the first minute or so of continuous high force isometric contractions. In everyday life, however, most activities, such as walking or running, involve either shortening or lengthening of the muscles, and tend to be repetitive.

8.6.1 *Changes during prolonged repetitive activity*

Prolonged, submaximal rhythmic exercises such as walking or running, during which muscles generate relatively low forces and there is sufficient time between contractions for substantial metabolic recovery, are common in everyday life. Central fatigue probably plays an important role in limiting performance during this type of activity with signals from skin, joint and tendon receptors feeding back to the central nervous system. In addition, core temperature, dehydration, altered blood electrolytes, hypoglycaemia and cerebral hypoxia will all affect motivation and central drive acting through both conscious and unconscious mechanisms.

There are also changes in muscle contractility associated with prolonged activity which cannot easily be ascribed to metabolic changes in the muscle. Such changes have been described in a number of different preparations and circumstances resulting in the condition generally known as *low-frequency fatigue* or LFF (Edwards *et al*, 1977).

After a long series of contractions there is generally a greater loss of force generated at lower, compared to higher, frequencies (Fig. 8.15) and a notable feature of this form of fatigue is that the recovery is slow occurring in hours and, on occasions, days.

During LFF the relatively normal force generated by high

frequencies of stimulation indicates that the contractile proteins retain their ability to generate force. It has been found that the muscle action potential remains normal and that the phosphocreatine and ATP content are restored to normal levels at times when low-frequency force is still reduced.

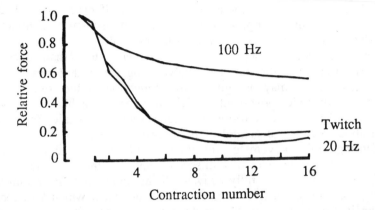

Fig. 8.15 Peak tension developed by a twitch and 1s tetani at 20 and 100Hz tested at intervals during a long series of ischaemic contractions. Results expressed as a fraction of the initial force showing greater loss of force at low frequencies than at high frequency (Edwards *et al*, 1977).

Experiments with isolated animal muscles have shown that the effects of LFF can be reversed by caffeine, further emphasising the fact that the defect is of the processes of activation, rather than of the function of the contractile proteins. This type of change in the contractile properties of the muscle may be due to a change in either the quantity of calcium released from the sarcoplasmic reticulum in response to a single action potential or in the affinity of troponin for calcium. Both of these defects would reduce the twitch force, while at higher frequencies when the interior of the fibre is saturated with calcium, relatively normal force would be produced.

It has been a frequent observation that LFF is more pronounced in muscles that have been exercised eccentrically (i.e. stretched when activated) than during either isometric or shortening contractions. Thus during stepping exercise, LFF is more pronounced in the quadriceps used to support the body whilst stepping down (eccentric contractions), despite the fact that these contractions are metabolically less demanding than the shortening (concentric) contractions of the opposite muscle used to step up.

This form of exercise is often accompanied by delayed onset pain and evidence of muscle damage in the form of release of soluble enzymes (see Chapter 9, Section 9.3.1). For these reasons, as well as the fact that it recovers so slowly, LFF has been thought to be a consequence of damage caused by the high forces generated in active muscle fibres rather than metabolic depletion.

8.6.2 *Dynamic exercise*

There is little information about how fatigue affects force production during movement as opposed to during an isometric contraction. Anecdotal reports of fatigue during running and cycling indicate that dynamic performance decreases to a greater extent than does the isometric strength of the muscles involved, suggesting that measurement of isometric force may not give a true reflection of the loss of force during the dynamic movements which make up most of our everyday activities. As with other forms of fatigue, loss of dynamic force could come about because of central or peripheral changes.

During rapid movements the duration of the contraction may be little more than a few tens of milliseconds and it is questionable whether this is sufficient time to fully activate all the motor units in the muscle. During shortening, muscle spindles will be unloaded which will reduce the excitatory inputs to the motoneurones. Despite the potential importance of central fatigue during dynamic movements involved in sporting activities, the phenomenon has not been systematically investigated.

8.6.2.1 *Peripheral changes leading to a loss of power*   There is evidence from animal muscle preparations that there are peripheral changes during dynamic contractions. An alteration in the shape of the force-velocity relationship is seen with fatigue, the main change being a reduction in the maximum velocity of shortening (Fig. 8.16). Consequently there is a proportionately greater loss of force the higher the velocities of shortening. The optimum velocity for maximum power output is reduced in the fatigued muscle as is both the maximum power itself and the power at any given velocity of shortening.

A change in the force-velocity relationship of a muscle implies a change in the kinetics of the cross-bridge interactions, probably involving slower rates of both attachment and detachment. It is not known what causes the change in cross-bridge cycling. It could be some covalent modification of the myosin (or less likely the actin) molecule such as the phosphorylation or dephosphorylation of one of the myosin light chains. Alternatively there may be some competition or influence of metabolites such as Pi or H^+ on the cross-bridge cycle, but, as discussed above in connection with the slowing of relaxation, changes in ATP or ADP are probably not large enough to affect directly the kinetics of the cross-bridge.

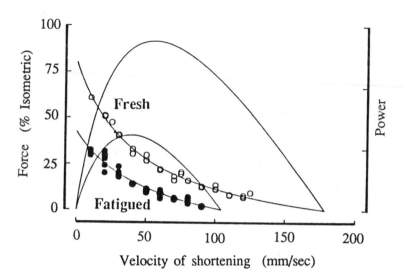

Fig. 8.16   Force-velocity relationships for fresh and fatigued muscles.   Rat gastrocnemius muscle. Data for fresh muscles (open symbols) and muscles after a 15s fatiguing tetanus (filled symbols; de Haan *et al*, 1989).

8.7 Summary

It will have become apparent that the two questions raised in the first paragraph of this chapter concerning the site of fatigue and its immediate cause have not been fully answered. This continuing uncertainty should not be surprising, considering the complexity of the neuromuscular system and the degree of integration required to produce a useful movement.   The best information that can be offered is that fatigue probably differs in its nature and cause depending on the type of exercise.

8.8 References and further reading

Bigland-Ritchie, B., Dawson, N.J., Johansson, R.S. & Lippold, O.C.J. (1986). Reflex origin for the slowing of motoneurone firing rates in fatigue of human voluntary contractions. *Journal of Physiology* **379**, 451-9.

Bigland-Ritchie, B., Jones, D.A., Hosking, G.P. & Edwards, R.H.T. (1978). Central and peripheral fatigue in sustained voluntary contractions of human quadriceps muscle. *Clinical Science* **54**, 609-14.

Bigland-Ritchie, B., Jones, D.A., Woods, J.J. (1979). Excitation frequency and muscle fatigue: electrical responses during voluntary and stimulated contractions. *Experimental Neurology* **64**, 414-27.

Bigland-Ritchie, B., Kukulka, C.G., Lippold, O.C.J. & Woods, J.J. (1982). The absence of neuromuscular junction transmission failure in sustained maximal voluntary contractions. *Journal of Physiology* **330**, 265-78.

Cady, E.B., Jones, D.A., Lynn, J. & Newham, D.J. (1989a). Changes in force and intracellular metabolites during fatigue of human skeletal muscle. *Journal of Physiology* **418**, 311-25.

Cady, E.B., Elshove, H., Jones, D.A. & Moll, A. (1989b). The metabolic causes of slow relaxation in fatigued human skeletal muscle. *Journal of Physiology* **418**, 327-37.

Cooke, R. & Bialek, W. (1979). Contraction of glycerinated muscle fibres as a function of MgATP concentration. *Biophysical Journal* **28**, 241-58.

Cooke, R. & Pate, E. (1985). The effects of ADP and phosphate on the contraction of muscle fibres. *Biophysical Journal* **48**, 789-98.

Crow, M.T. & Kushmerick, M.J. (1983). Correlated reduction in velocity of shortening and rate of energy utilization in mouse fast-twitch muscle during a continuous tetanus. *Journal of General Physiology* **82**, 703-20.

Dawson, M.J., Gadian, D.G. & Wilkie, D.R. (1978). Muscular fatigue investigated by phosphorous nuclear magnetic resonance. *Nature* **274**, 861-6.

de Haan, A., Jones, D.A. & Sargeant, A.J. (1989). Changes in velocity of shortening, power output and relaxation rate during fatigue of rat medial gastrocnemius muscle. *Pflügers Archiv* **413**, 422-8.

Donaldson, S.K.B. & Hermansen, L. (1978). Differential, direct effects of H^+ on Ca^{2+}-activated force of skinned fibres from soleus, cardiac and adductor magnus muscles of rabbits. *Pflügers Archiv* **376**, 55-65.

Edwards, R.H.T., Hill, D.K. & Jones, D.A. (1975). Metabolic changes associated with slowing of relaxation in fatigued mouse muscle. *Journal of Physiology* **251**, 287-301.

Edwards, R.H.T., Hill, D.K., Jones, D.A. & Merton, P.A. (1977). Fatigue of long duration in human muscle after exericise. *Journal of Physiology* **272**, 769-78.

Fabiato, A. & Fabiato, F. (1978). Effects of pH on the myofilaments and the sarcoplasmic reticulum of skinned cells from cardiac and skeletal muscles. *Journal of Physiology* **276**, 233-55.

Hnik, P., Holas, M., Krekule, I., Mejsnar, J., Smiesko, V., Ujec, E. & Vyskocil, F. (1976). Work-induced potassium changes in skeletal muscle and effluent venous blood assessed by liquid ion-exchanger microelectrodes. *Pflügers Archiv* **362**, 84-95.

Jones, D.A. & Bigland-Ritchie, B. (1986). Electrical and contractile changes in muscle fatigue. In: *Biochemistry of Exercise VI,* ed. B. Saltin. International Series on Sports Sciences, Vol 16. Champaign, Ill., Human Kinetics Publishers. pp. 377-92.

Jones, D.A., Bigland-Ritchie, B. & Edwards, R.H.T. (1979). Excitation frequency and muscle fatigue: mechanical responses during voluntary and stimulated contractions. *Experimental Neurology* **64**, 401-13.

Kentish, J.C. (1986). The effects of inorganic phosphate and creatine phosphate on force production in skinned muscles from rat ventricle. *Journal of Physiology* **370**, 585-604.

Krnjevic, K. & Miledi, R. (1958). Failure of neuromuscular propagation in rats. *Journal of Physiology* **140**, 440-61.

Lannergren, J. & Westerblad, H. (1986). Force and membrane potential during and after fatiguing, continuous high frequency stimulation of single *Xenopus* muscle fibres. *Acta Physiologica Scandinavia* **128**, 359-68.

Lannergren, J. & Westerblad, H. (1987). Action potential fatigue in single skeletal muscle fibres of *Xenopus*. *Acta Physiologica Scandinavia* **129**, 311-18.

Merton, P.A. (1954). Voluntary strength and fatigue. *Journal of Physiology.* **123**, 553-64.

Nosek, T.M., Fender, K.Y. & Godt, R.E. (1987). It is diprotonated inorganic phosphate that depresses force in skinned skeletal muscle fibres. *Science* **236**, 191-3.

Sjogaard, G., Adams, R.P. & Saltin, B. (1985). Water and ion shifts in skeletal muscle of humans with intense dynamic knee extension. *American Journal of Physiology* **248**, R190-6.

Stephens, J.A. & Taylor, A. (1972). Fatigue of voluntary muscle contractions in man. *Journal of Physiology* **220**, 1-18.

Chapter 9

MUSCLE DAMAGE

Muscles may be damaged in a number of ways: as a result of physical trauma, as a consequence of excessive use or due to some pathological process. In this chapter we will review the various causes of damage and then go on to consider the sequel to damage in healthy muscle, namely repair and regeneration.

9.1 Physical trauma

By the nature of their position in the body, skeletal muscles are frequently subjected to physical trauma and this risk is increased with participation in contact sports. There is little information about the extent of muscle fibre damage which occurs as a result of the bumps and bruises of everyday life, but probably most of the painful sensations experienced are due to inflammation of the skin, subcutaneous tissue and muscle fascia, with relatively little involvement of the muscle fibres. Where there is major disruption of the tissue, muscle may be replaced with scar tissue.

After severe crush injuries or if an unconscious person has been lying undiscovered on a hard surface for several hours, myoglobinuria may be present. Myoglobin in the urine is clear evidence of muscle fibre damage and is a serious complication, not so much because of the muscle damage, but because myoglobin tends to precipitate in the kidneys, leading to renal failure. Muscle damage can be conveniently monitored by measuring intracellular components released into the blood. The most commonly estimated proteins are myoglobin and the enzymes creatine kinase (CK), lactate dehydrogenase (LDH) and aspartate transaminase. The advantage of measuring CK and LDH is that they have muscle-specific isoenzymic forms which allows effluxes from skeletal muscle to be distinguished from enzyme coming from cardiac muscle or other tissue.

Peripheral nerves are susceptible to physical damage. Degeneration of a motor axon leads to denervation of the motor unit followed by re-innervation by surviving intact axons. Repeated peripheral nerve damage will lead to a loss of fine motor control as motor units are lost to be replaced with fewer and larger units.

9.2 **Metabolic depletion**

Large metabolic fluxes occur during intense exercise and it is natural to wonder whether excessive metabolic depletion leads to long-lasting change in muscle which might be classified as "damage".

9.2.1 *Isolated muscle preparations*

9.2.1.1 *Calcium entry and fibre damage*   Metabolic depletion can be produced in isolated mouse muscle preparations by prolonged electrical stimulation or the addition of poisons such as cyanide, dinitrophenol or iodoacetic acid (Jones *et al*, 1983). This treatment leads to the release of LDH into the bathing medium which reaches a peak 30 to 60 minutes after the metabolic insult (Fig. 9.1).

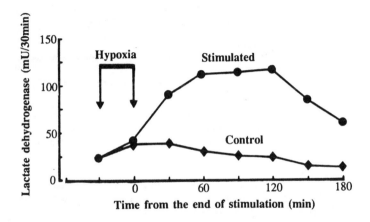

Fig. 9.1 Enzyme release from mouse soleus muscles. Muscles were hypoxic during the 30 minutes indicated, during which time half the muscles were stimulated.

The damaged muscles have raised intracellular calcium concentrations and the damage can be largely prevented by withdrawing external calcium from the bathing medium (Jones *et al*, 1984; Fig. 9.2). These findings suggest that the entry of calcium into muscle cells is involved in the initiation of damage, a theory which is supported by the fact that muscle preparations incubated in A23187, a calcium ionophore which allows the movement of calcium into cells, also leads to an efflux of soluble muscle constituents followed by structural damage to the cell. In a healthy fibre there is about a one thousandfold concentration gradient of calcium across the surface membrane, consequently small changes in calcium permeability will result in a rapid influx; how calcium permeability is regulated by internal metabolite concentrations is not known but it has been shown that depletion of ATP or PC clearly allows calcium entry. It is not known whether calcium enters through regular calcium ion channels or through disruptions in the surface membrane.

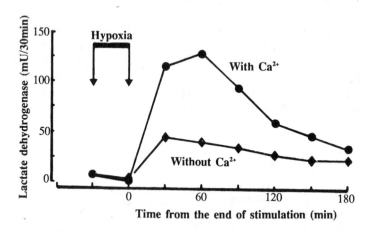

Fig. 9.2 The effect of external calcium on the release of enzymes from isolated mouse soleus muscles. All muscles were stimulated during the hypoxic period. In one set of muscles the medium was calcium free from the start of the stimulation and for the remainder of the experiment.

Many poisons have the entry of calcium as a final common step in the sequence of events leading to cell death (Schanne *et al*, 1979). Once inside the cell, calcium ions can have a number of deleterious actions. Within the muscle fibre there is a protease and a phospholipase, both of which are calcium-activated enzymes, which could cause severe damage to the structure of the muscle fibre. In mouse muscle preparations, inhibitors of calcium-activated proteases such as leupeptin and pepstatin do not prevent muscle cell damage caused by metabolic depletion. However some inhibitors of the calcium activated phospholipase such as dibucaine, mepacrine and chlorpromazine substantially reduce the enzyme efflux (Jackson *et al*, 1984), suggesting an important role for this enzyme in the degregative process. The activated phospholipase liberates free fatty acids from membrane-bound triglycerides, a process which may directly affect the structure of cell membranes. In addition, the free fatty acids liberated in the process could have a detergent action causing further damage to membranes both of the cell wall and of intracellular organelles (Fig. 9.3). Among the fatty acids liberated is arachidonic acid which can be converted to biologically active compounds by cyclo-oxygenase or lipoxygenase enzymes. Cyclo-oxygenase inhibitors have no effect on enzyme release from damaged muscle but some lipoxygenase inhibitors are very effective in preventing release (Jackson *et al*, 1987). These findings suggest that it is not the primary action of phospholipase that is damaging so much as the subsequent metabolism of the liberated free fatty acids.

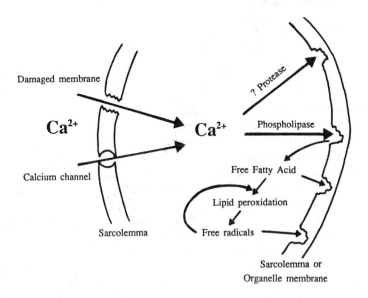

Fig. 9.3 Suggested mechanisms of muscle damage. Calcium entry may activate phospholipases and, possibly, protease enzymes. The free fatty acids liberated will, in turn, have a detergent effect on cell membranes and may be the substrate for free radical attack.

Although phospholipase inhibitors provide some protection against structural damage and the release of enzymes, they do not protect against the loss of function in the metabolically depleted muscles.

9.2.1.2 *Free radical damage* Free fatty acids are readily oxidised within cells and, in the process, can generate free radicals. Free radicals are highly reactive species which can initiate a chain reaction leading to the oxidation of other lipids and the disruption of cell membranes. Free radical mediated damage is thought to be a major cause of the reperfusion injury of cardiac muscle where damage and enzyme release is initiated, not by ischaemia but by the restoration of an oxygenated circulation (Guarnieri *et al*, 1978). A similar mechanism could exist in skeletal muscle but evidence that this occurs as a result of exercise remains circumstantial. Vitamin E is a natural antioxidant that can reduce free radical reactions in muscle homogenates, but adding vitamin E to the incubation system illustrated in Fig. 9.1 provides no protective effect and does not reduce the enzyme efflux. However, a comparison of muscles from mice maintained on a vitamin E deficient diet with muscles from animals on the same diet but supplemented with vitamin E, showed the deficient muscles to be more susceptible to damage caused by metabolic depletion (Jackson *et al*, 1983).

9.2.1.3 *Summary of the mechanisms of damage* There are three aspects of the mechanism causing the type of damage associated with metabolic depletion. The first is calcium entry consequent upon a change in muscle metabolite levels (a decrease in ATP or increase in ADP, etc.). The second aspect is the intracellular action of calcium in stimulating phospholipase thereby causing damage to cellular membranes, while the third element is free radical damage initiated by the oxidation of the liberated free fatty acids. A number of compounds can protect against the damage which occurs as a result of metabolic depletion, and these may act on specific sites (e.g. phospholipase inhibitors, vitamin E and free radicals scavengers). However most of the protective agents have more than one possible mode of action and many of the phospholipase inhibitors are also local anaesthetics. Vitamin E, the phospholipase inhibitors and the lipoxygenase inhibitiors are lipid soluble and there is a suspicion that, in addition to their supposed specific action, these agents may have a general membrane stabilising effect, dissolving in the membrane lipid layer and altering the conformation of the surface membrane to make it less susceptible to attack by phospholipase or free radicals.

9.2.2 *Muscle damage during fatiguing exercise*
There is little evidence that conventional exercise testing, such as work on a cycle ergometer or treadmill, leads to any significant muscle damage. Heavy exercise of this type, maintained for an hour or so, can result in a doubling of the circulating CK, which reaches a peak about 24 hours after the exercise with a return to normal levels within 48 hours. The possibility has been explored that patients with various muscle disorders may have their condition exacerbated by exercise or that a subclinical or carrier state might be revealed as an abnormal response to a standard exercise protocol (Brooke *et al*, 1979). Although some abnormalities were found, the most striking feature was that conventional hard work, such as running uphill or working against a high load on a cycle ergometer, produces very little evidence of muscle damage.

Long-lasting fatigue can be produced in single human muscle groups by repeated high-force contractions (see Chapter 8, Section 8.13) and the changes can take as long as 24 to 48 hours to fully recover, which suggests there may have been some form of damage. However, this form of fatigue, which characteristically affects force production at low frequencies more than at high, is unlikely to be a consequence of metabolic depletion within the muscle as it is most evident as a result of exercise in which the active muscle is stretched and where the metabolic costs are relatively low (see below). Periods of ischaemia lasting an hour or so are often used to create a bloodless field to work in during orthopaedic surgery or operations on the hand and must result in metabolic depletion, but the muscle appears to be relatively unaffected by such procedures.

9.2.2.1 *Muscle damage and exercise in disease* It seems unlikely that the metabolite changes which occur in normal muscle as a result of exercise are ever sufficient to result in the type of damage that can be produced in isolated preparations by prolonged stimulation under anaerobic conditions or treatment with metabolic inhibitors. There are, however, some rare pathological conditions in which metabolic depletion can lead to severe damage, probably by the mechanism suggested for the isolated muscle preparations. One such condition is malignant hyperpyrexia (see Chapter 11, Section 11.12), in which skeletal muscle responds to the anaesthetic halothane with a prolonged contracture causing metabolic depletion of the muscle. The first sign of danger is a rise in body temperature and release of potassium into the circulation which brings with it the risk of cardiac arrest. If the patient survives the acute emergency much of the skeletal muscle subsequently undergoes necrosis releasing a mass of soluble proteins including myoglobin which, in turn, can lead to renal failure and another life-threatening crisis. A similar condition exists in some breeds of pig where stress can also be a precipitating factor.

A similar sequence of events, rigor followed by muscle fibre necrosis, can occur in patients with defects of the glycolytic pathway, for example in myophosphorylase or phosphofructokinase deficiency, if prolonged vigorous muscular activity is undertaken. Fortunately, these patients are usually well aware of their limitations and take care to reduce their exercise before any crisis can develop.

Patients with defective mitochondrial function might be expected to have similar problems but, in practice, they do not present with muscle damage following exercise. Although often severely limited in their exercise capacity, the normal glycolytic function in these patients must provide sufficient energy to prevent their muscles going into contracture.

Patients with disorders of fatty acid metabolism often report episodes of muscle pain and myoglobinuria. While exercise may sometimes be the precipitating factor, infections or alcohol are often also implicated.

It is unlikely that metabolic depletion is the cause of the muscle damage in these patients and it is possible that high levels of free fatty acids may be the immediate cause. Exercise mobilises free fatty acids from body fat depots and muscle triglycerides but, because in these patients, fatty acid transport into the mitochondria is defective, the free fatty acids will accumulate within the muscle fibre. The majority of fatty acids in the body are stearic and palmitic acids; stearic acid is the principal component of domestic soap and can have a damaging detergent action on cell membranes.

There are frequent reports of young recruits in the armed forces who collapse complaining of muscle pain after route marches or similar intensive exercise. These individuals often pass dark urine containing myoglobin, suggesting that muscle damage has occurred. Very occasionally the problem is found to be a defect of glycolysis, but the majority of cases remain undiagnosed. It is possible that in some cases the unaccustomed heavy exercise has revealed a subclinical defect of fatty acid metabolism of the type discussed above.

There has been considerable interest in the possibility that vitamin E deficiency may lead to free radical induced muscle damage. A condition known as "white muscle disease" occurs in cattle that have been kept indoors over winter eating feeds low in vitamin E. On being released into the fields in spring the animals suffer from muscle degeneration, possibly associated with unaccustomed activity (Allen *et al*, 1975). The condition is readily prevented by injections of vitamin E and selenium. Selenium is an essential component of the enzyme superoxide dismutase, important for removing free radicals. Despite the veterinary evidence there has been no convincing demonstration of any association between vitamin E deficiency and human muscle damage. Trials of vitamin E as a treatment for Duchenne muscular dystrophy have proved unrewarding (Edwards *et al*, 1984).

9.3 Damage due to eccentric contractions

During metabolically demanding exercise such as cycling or running on the level or uphill, the major muscle groups are shortening whilst active and this form of muscular activity is sometimes known as "concentric exercise" or "positive work". Another type of muscular activity, which is equally common and just as important, is where muscles are used to support a weight, either the body or some external load, as this is lowered such as lifting objects off a high shelf, walking downstairs or when sitting down. During these movements the active muscles are stretched and in so doing can generate high forces, nearly twice that of an isometric contraction and, depending on the speed, several times more than during shortening, concentric contractions (Chapter 2, Section 2.4.4).

During everyday life this fact presents no problem but if the exercise is unfamiliar or particularly vigorous, delayed onset muscle pain and tenderness are an unpleasant consequence (Chapter 10, Section 10.3.1). During the conventional Harvard step test, in which a subject steps on and off a bench, one leg is used to step up and the other to support the weight of the body during the downward step. During the step up the quadriceps and gluteal muscles of the stepping leg shorten (concentric contractions) while during the step down the same muscles of the other leg are stretched whilst under tension (eccentric contractions).

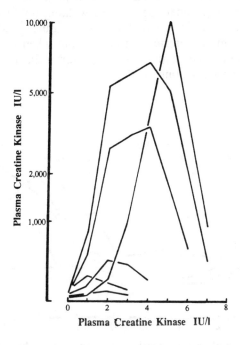

Fig. 9.4   Plasma creatine kinase levels following 30 minutes stepping exercise. Subjects stepped on and off a stool adjusted to just above knee height at a frequency of 15 cycles a minute using, every time, the same leg to step up and the opposite to step down.

If this test is prolonged for about 30 minutes, always with the same leg stepping down, most subjects develop considerable pain and stiffness in the muscle used to step down 24 to 48 hours later and about half show a delayed rise in plasma CK. There is little change in the circulating level of CK during the first 48 hours but 4 to 5 days after the exercise many subjects have a very large response with up to a hundredfold increase in plasma levels (Fig. 9.4; Newham *et al*, 1983). If the circumstances were not known the high circulating levels of CK would suggest a severe degenerative muscle disease.

It is not known why some people are more susceptible than others to this form of damage. It may be, in part, a training effect (see below, Section 9.3.3), but experience shows that there is a wide variation in muscle response to eccentric exercise which is not related to general fitness, age or sex.

The development of muscle pain in the leg used to step down leads to the assumption that the CK appearing in the blood has come from damaged muscle in that leg. However this assumption requires some proof because the CK has been released into the general circulation and could have come from either leg. When walking uphill on an inclined treadmill the major muscle groups (quadriceps, gluteal and calf muscles) shorten and perform concentric contractions but when the subjects walk *backwards* downhill the same muscle groups will be stretched and perform eccentric contractions.

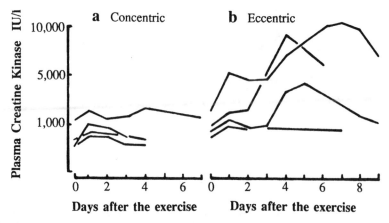

Fig. 9.5 Changes in plasma creatine kinase following treadmill exercise. a, subjects walked up an inclined treadmill. b, subjects walked backwards down the same incline. In b the exercise stretched the active calf and gluteal muscles.

Following this type of protocol, and with subjects walking uphill, a small rise in CK is seen at 24 hours after exercise (Fig. 9.5a), much as has been reported for other forms of vigorous exercise involving concentric contractions. For the subjects walking downhill there is a similar rise in CK at 24 hours followed, in most cases, by a very large rise 4 to 5 days later. These results clearly demonstrate that it is the eccentric exercise that results in muscle damage and the delayed release of CK. This large rise in circulating CK has been shown to be due to a raised muscle CK fraction, and is therefore not due to damage to cardiac muscle.

The release of CK represents an increased permeability of the muscle cell membrane and is mirrored by an increased uptake of radioactive tracer (e.g. technicium pyrophosphate) into the exercised muscles.

Muscle biopsies taken from exercised muscles, both immediately after exercise and 24 hours later, show little evidence of damage when examined by light microscopy. At the EM level some evidence of structural damage, for example Z line streaming, can be seen (Fridén *et al*, 1983: Newham *et al*, 1983). If the muscle is biopsied a few days after the peak of circulating CK, muscle fibre necrosis, inflammatory mononuclear cell invasions of the muscle and fibre regeneration are all apparent.

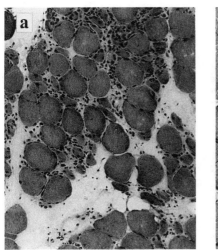 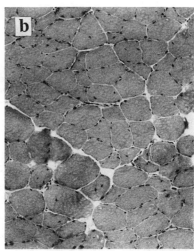

Fig. 9.6 The appearance of muscle biopsy specimens taken from a calf muscle **a**, 12 and **b**, 20 days after eccentric exercise (stained with H&E).

In some cases the extent of the fibre damage can be large, with up to 50% of fibres in a biopsy specimen affected (Jones *et al*, 1986). Further biopsies show that regeneration is virtually complete 3 to 4 weeks after the damaging exercise (Fig. 9.6).

The microscopic appearance of the damaged muscle is very similar to that seen in the severe inflammatory myopathies such as polymyositis.

The same patterns of cellular infiltration are seen as are the types of infiltrating cells, which are mainly macrophages and include both T helper and T suppressor cells, but not B cells or NK cells (Round *et al*, 1987). The difference between the experimental damage and the disease is that the normal subjects recover within a few weeks but polymyositis has a poor prognosis. The pathogenesis of polymyositis is unknown, there being a debate as to whether there is an abnormality in the immune system which provokes an attack on otherwise healthy muscle or whether the muscle is abnormal, perhaps expressing unusual surface antigens as a result of viral infection, the cellular infiltration being a normal response of the immune system to abnormal muscle. The appearance of the experimentally damaged muscle suggests that the cellular infiltration seen in the inflammatory myopathies is a normal response to an abnormal muscle, thus puting the emphasis on an abnormality of muscle as being the primary cause of the disorder.

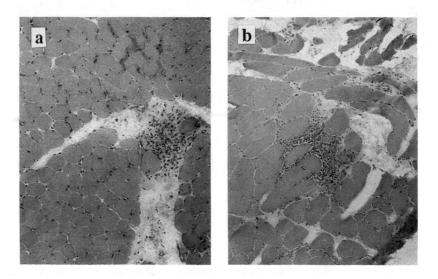

Fig. 9.7   Cellular infiltration in damaged muscle. **a**, Human biceps 10 days after eccentric exercise. **b**, female patient (45 years) with polymyositis. (H&E stain).

9.3.1   *Changes in muscle force after eccentric exercise*

Following 20 to 30 minutes of rhythmic exercise such as stepping on and off a box the quadriceps muscle that has been stretched while active is found to have lost more force at the end of exercise than the opposite muscle that has been shortening while stepping up. Not only is the maximum force generated by the stretched muscle reduced, but there are also changes in the force-frequency relationship such that relatively less force is generated at low frequencies of stimulation, being the same phenomenon as the low-frequency fatigue (LFF) discussed in Chapter 8 (Section 8.6.1). The loss of force is greatest immediately after exercise and can persist for several days, slowly returning to normal over one or two weeks (Newham *et al*, 1987). Changes in the force-frequency curve are maximal immediately after the exercise and also recover with a slow time course (Fig. 9.8). Although high forces are generated when an active muscle is stretched, they are produced at a low metabolic cost (Chapter 2, Section 2.4.5).

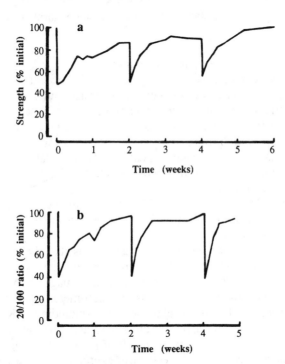

Fig. 9.8 Biceps muscle strength (**a**) and contractile properties (**b**) following bouts of eccentric exercise repeated at intervals of two weeks. Note that training has no protective effect on the force loss immediately after the exercise. The contractile properties (**b**) are expressed as the ratio of force generated at low (20Hz) compared to high frequency (100Hz) stimulation.

Since LFF is greatest in muscles that have been exercising eccentrically it would appear that this form of fatigue is unlikely to be caused by metabolic depletion and is certainly not due to persisting muscle acidosis, or other metabolic change, since the muscle metabolites are restored to normal within minutes at the end of exercise whereas LFF can persist for many hours. The alternative explanation is that these changes in contractile properties are due to damage occurring as a result of the high forces generated in the muscle. It has been found that the changes are greatest if the muscle is exercised at a long length (Jones *et al*, 1989). At long muscle fibre lengths differences in sarcomere length along the fibre lead to the phenomenon of "creep" (see Chapter 2, Section 2.2) whereby the shorter, stronger sarcomeres at the ends of a fibre pull out the sarcomeres in the centre. During eccentric contractions this pulling out of the central sarcomeres could be accentuated to the extent of causing structural damage to the fibre. There is, as yet, no explanation as to how such damage might give rise to LFF.

9.3.2 *The time course of muscle damage*

A major feature of the damage caused by eccentric contractions is the delay of several days between the exercise and the massive release of CK from the muscle. The appearance in the general circulation of substances released from any tissue may be delayed by diffusion and mixing within the lymphatic system. The various enzymes released from a damaged heart reach a peak in the circulation in a matter of hours after the infarct. Similar considerations of diffusion and drainage could account for the peak CK occurring at 24 hours after heavy exercise involving concentric contractions but they cannot account for the delay of several days before CK is released from muscle damaged by eccentric contractions.

The implication of the delayed response is that the exercise initiates a sequence of events which results in gross damage several days later. In the early stages, the only visible signs of damage to muscle fibres are areas of Z-line streaming and loss of sarcomere structure. The next event is release of intracellular proteins (including CK) and this is followed by degeneration of muscle fibres and infiltration of the tissue by mononuclear cells (Jones *et al*, 1986). One interpretation of this sequence of events is that the eccentric exercise causes a certain amount of structural damage to the muscle fibre, probably accounting for the loss of force and changes in contractile properties. If this damage is not adequately repaired within a day or so the fibre, or at least a segment of the fibre, degenerates, releasing soluble proteins into the circulation. The infiltration of macrophages and T cells is a process of removing cellular debris and initiating regeneration. The extent of these changes is modified by training.

9.3.3 *The effect of training*

If subjects are trained by repeated bouts of eccentric exercise there is a very marked change in the pain experienced and the amount of muscle damage estimated by the appearance of CK in the plasma (Fig. 9.9). The protection afforded by a single bout of eccentric exercise lasts for between 6 and 12 weeks but the mechanism responsible for the increased resistance is not known. One explanation of the training effect is that the muscle becomes less susceptible to the structural damage that may initiate the sequence of events described above. It is particularly noticeable, however, that repeated exercise, whilst protecting the muscle against the fibre degeneration that leads to the loss of creatine kinase, does not result in any change in susceptibility of the muscle to loss of force or change in contractile characteristics (Fig. 9.8). If the loss of force and change in contractile properties represent the start of the sequence of events leading to fibre degeneration, then the training adaptation must be such that it enhances the extent to which this damage can be repaired thus breaking the downward spiral towards muscle fibre death.

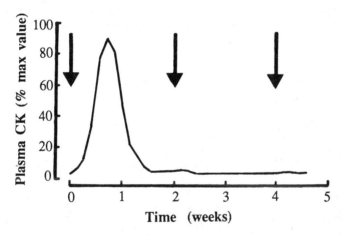

Fig. 9.9 Plasma creatine kinase following eccentric exercise. The exercise was repeated at the start of weeks 2 and 4. The values are expressed as a percentage of the highest value recorded after the first bout of exercise.

9.4 Muscle regeneration

There has been a widespread belief that skeletal muscle does not regenerate after injury but it is now clear that, on the contrary, it possesses considerable powers of regeneration. Among the pioneers in this field was Studitsky (1964) who showed that a muscle that was removed, minced and then returned to the original site surprisingly regenerated into a functional muscle. A similar picture of degeneration followed by regeneration is seen if a muscle is damaged *in situ*, either by crushing, making it ischaemic or exercising with eccentric contractions. The extent of regeneration depends on the degree to which the basement membranes of the original fibres have been preserved and whether the tracts of the nerves and blood vessels to the transplant area remain intact (see Carlson & Faulkner, 1983, for a review of the subject).

Muscles which have been removed, minced and replaced are the least successful at regenerating, recovering to about one-quarter to half the former size and strength. If the muscle is taken out and the nerves and blood vessels severed, the extent of regeneration will be limited by the success of the regrowth of nerves and blood vessels. Muscles that have been caused to degenerate by occlusion of the blood supply or by the use of myotoxins give the best results as the connective tissue architecture of the muscle remains intact. The basement membranes of the original fibres act as a guide within which myoblasts can develop and fuse to form new fibres. Similarly nerve and blood vessel regeneration is far more succesful if they can grow along the track of the degenerate nerve or blood vessel. In this situation anastomosing cut ends of nerves and blood vessels by microsurgery increases both the speed and extent of the regrowth.

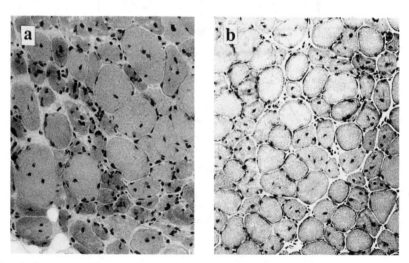

Fig. 9.10 Regeneration following damage by eccentric exercise. Mouse anterior tibialis. **a**, five days after damage showing the formation of myoblasts. **b**, twenty days after damage showing a range of fibre sizes and central nuclei.

Regeneration follows a number of stages; the first is autolysis, where all structure is apparently lost, followed by invasion of the necrotic mass by blood vessels. Mononuclear cells, including macrophages and T lymphocytes, move from the blood vessels and infiltrate the tissue. This phase is associated with the division of surviving satellite cells, their maturation into myoblasts and fusion to form new myotubes (Fig. 9.10a). After this stage the maturation and innervation of the new muscle probably proceeds by the same sequence of events as occurs in the embryo. A crucial, but poorly understood, stage in regeneration is the stimulation of satellite cells to divide. Invasion of the necrotic mass by macrophages seems to be an essential prerequisite for regeneration and it is possible that the invading mononuclear cells may produce factors which stimulate satellite cell division.

Although substantial regeneration occurs, the new muscle often has a wider range of fibre sizes than the original muscle and central nuclei are a prominent feature which can remain for a long time (Fig. 9.10b).

Muscle fibres are long multinucleate cells and it is not clear whether damage to a discrete area, say in the middle, leads to the degeneration of the whole fibre. It seems likely that in many situations the damage can be contained and localised with satellite cells replacing only the damaged portions.

9.5 References and further reading

Allen, W.M., Bradley, R., Berrett, S., Par, W.H., Swannack, K., Barton, C.R.O. & MacPhee, A. (1975). Degenerative myopathy with myoglobinuria in yearling cattle. *British Veterinary Journal* **131**, 292-308.

Brooke, M.H., Carroll, J.E., Davis, J.E. & Hagberg, J.M. (1979). The prolonged exercise test. *Neurology* **29**, 636-43.

Carlson, B.M. & Faulkner, J.A. (1983). The regeneration of skeletal muscle fibres following injury: a review. *Medicine & Science in Sports & Exercise* **15**, 187-98.

Edwards, R.H.T., Jones, D.A. & Jackson, M.J. (1984). An approach to treatment trials in muscular dystrophy with particular reference to agents influencing free radical damage. *Medical Biology* **62**, 143-47.

Fridén, J., Sjostrom, M. & Ekblom, B. (1983). Myofibrillar damage following intense eccentric exercise in man. *International Journal of Sports Medicine* **4**, 170-6.

Guarnieri, C., Ferrari, R., Visioli, O., Caldarera, C.M. & Nayler, W.G. (1978). Effect of α-tocophorol on hypoxic-perfused and reoxygenated rabbit heart muscle. *Journal of Molecular and Cellular Cardiology* **10**, 893-906.

Jackson, M.J., Jones, D.A. & Edwards, R.H.T. (1983). Vitamin E and skeletal muscle. In: *Biology of Vitamin E* (Ciba Foundation symposium 101). London, Pitman Books, pp. 224-39.

Jackson, M.J., Jones, D.A. & Edwards, R.H.T. (1984). Experimental skeletal muscle damage: the nature of the calcium-activated degenerative process. *European Journal of Clinical Investigation* **14**, 369-74.

Jackson, M.J., Wagenmakers, J.M. & Edwards, R.H.T. (1987). Effect of inhibitors of arachidonic acid metabolism on efflux of intracellular enzymes from skeletal muscle following experimental damage. *Biochemical Journal* **241**, 403-7.

Jones, D.A., Jackson, M.J. & Edwards, R.H.T. (1983). Release of intracellular enzymes from an isolated mammalian skeletal muscle preparation. *Clinical Science* **65**, 193-201.

Jones, D.A., Jackson, M.J., McPhail, G. & Edwards, R.H.T. (1984). Experimental mouse muscle damage: the importance of external calcium. *Clinical Science* **66**, 317-22.

Jones, D.A., Newham, D.J., Round, J.M. & Tolfree, S.E.J. (1986). Experimental muscle damage: morphological changes in relation to other indices of damage. *Journal of Physiology* **375**, 435-48.

Jones, D.A., Newham, D.J. & Torgan, C. (1989). Mechanical influences on long-lasting human muscle fatigue and delayed onset pain. *Journal of Physiology* **412**, 415-27.

Newham, D.J., Jones, D.A. & Clarkson, P.M. (1987). Repeated high-force eccentric exercise: effects on muscle pain and damage. *Journal of Applied Physiology* **63**, 1381-6.

Newham, D.J., Jones, D.A. & Edwards, R.H.T. (1983). Large and delayed plasma creatine kinase changes after stepping exerise. *Muscle and Nerve* **6**, 36-41.

Newham, D.J., Jones, D.A. & Edwards, R.H.T. (1986). Plasma Creatine kinase after concentric and eccentric contractions. *Muscle and Nerve* **9**, 59-63.

Newham, D.J., McPhail, G., Mills, K.R. & Edwards, R.H.T. (1983). Ultrastructural changes after concentric and eccentric contractions of human muscle. *Journal of the Neurological Sciences* **61**, 109-22.

Newham, D.J., Mills, K.R., Quigley, B.M. & Edwards, R.H.T. (1983). Pain and fatigue following concentric and eccentric contractions. *Clinical Science* **64**, 55-62.

Round, J.M., Jones, D.A. & Cambridge, G. (1987). Cellular infiltrates in human skeletal muscle: exercise induced damage as a model for inflammatory muscle disease? *Journal of the Neurological Sciences* **82**, 1-11

Schanne, F., Kane, A.B., Young, E.E. & Farber, J.L. (1979). Calcium dependence of toxic cell death: a common final pathway. *Science* **206**, 700-2.

Studitsky, A.N. (1964). Free, auto and homografts of muscle tissue in experiments on animals. *Annals of the New York Academey of Science* **120**, 789-901.

Chapter 10

MUSCULAR PAIN

Muscular pain during and after exercise must be one of the most commonly experienced forms of discomfort yet relatively little is known about its causes. There are two main types of pain associated with exercise, one arising during the activity and the other of delayed onset, occurring some time afterwards and generally called "muscular stiffness" but often described in the literature as delayed onset muscle soreness (or DOMS, Armstrong, 1984). This chapter is concerned mainly with these two forms of muscular pain but will first deal briefly with the classification of sensory nerves and their endings and on methods of quantifying pain in human subjects. For a review of all aspects of pain, including a chapter on muscle, see Wall & Melzack (1989).

10.1 Sensory nerves

There are a variety of sensory nerve endings in muscle and their afferent nerves are categorised according to size, conduction velocity and whether or not they are myelinated. The sensations evoked by stimulation of the endings varies according to the type of nerve. The main types are given in Table 10.1.

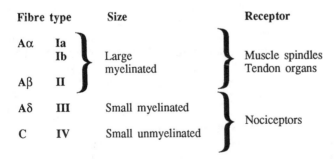

Fibre type		Size	Receptor
Aα	Ia	Large myelinated	Muscle spindles Tendon organs
	Ib		
Aβ	II		
Aδ	III	Small myelinated	Nociceptors
C	IV	Small unmyelinated	

Table 10.1 The classification of sensory nerve fibres.

The small myelinated (type III or Aδ) and unmyelinated (type IV or C) fibres are concerned with signalling pain. These nerves are freely branching in muscle and their unencapsulated endings are particularly dense in the myotendinous junctions and fascial sheaths. Stimulation of type III fibres gives rise to an immediate sensation of pain described as short-lasting, well localised and of a pinprick quality, whilst simulation of type IV fibres results in more diffuse pain, of longer duration and having a dull or burning quality.

Most muscle pain receptors are thought to be polymodal, that is they will respond to mechanical, thermal or chemical stimuli and one substance may potentiate, or lower the threshold, for another. This potentiation may be the mechanism underlying the development of tenderness where, under the influence of some chemical stimulus, the tissue becomes sensitive to a degree of pressure that would not normally produce any painful response. Substances known to excite receptors in muscle include bradykinin, serotonin, histamine, potassium, hypertonic saline and hydrogen ions.

10.1.1 *Quantification of pain*

To study and understand the nature of pain it is necessary to try and quantify the sensations but, in common with all other feelings, pain is a very subjective experience. With animal preparations it is often possible to record from the afferent nerve and obtain information about the characteristics of specific nerve endings by measuring firing frequencies in response to graded stimuli. With human subjects, however, this technique is not possible and experiments have to rely on some form of reporting of the perceived pain by the subject. The simplest way is to ask the subject to rate the discomfort on a scale of, say, 1 to 10. This method has two drawbacks: the first is that the divisions may be too wide to distinguish one level of pain from another. The second is that this method forces both subject and investigator to think in terms of a linear scale. The first problem can be circumvented, to some extent, by using an analogue scale with which the subject indicates the level of pain as the distance along a continuous line, one end of which represents no pain and the other unbearable pain. Towards the limits of pain a small increase in stimulus may double the sensation, yet the subject finds he has already rated the previous test as 9 on the scale of 1 to 10 and has no way of recording the full increase in pain.

A better way of recording pain is to use an open-ended scale in which the subject chooses any number to represent the pain associated with some intermediate level of stimulation and then scales all subsequent tests in relation to the initial reference stimulus. In this situation there is no upper limit and the reported pain often increases exponentially as the noxious stimulus approaches its maximum. Non-verbal ways of recording sensations have obvious advantages and can include moving a lever or turning a dial in response to increments of pain. Tenderness can be assessed by measuring the threshold pressure required to elicit a sensation of pain in the muscle (see Section 10.3.3).

Whatever method of measurement is used, it is evident that the reporting of pain is always subjective and the perception of a noxious stimulus can differ greatly between people and may also vary with the person's mood, health or hormonal status.

10.2 Muscle pain during activity

10.2.1 *Experimental studies of normal subjects*
During high-intensity exercise such as running up a long flight of stairs, discomfort develops rapidly in the working muscles. Although specific mechanisms have still to be identified, the general nature of the processes involved and the origin of the pain-producing substance can be inferred from a number of simple observations on muscle, working with and without an intact circulation. Most physical exercise uses large muscle groups but the general mechanisms involved can be more conveniently investigated using the small muscles of the hand and forearm.

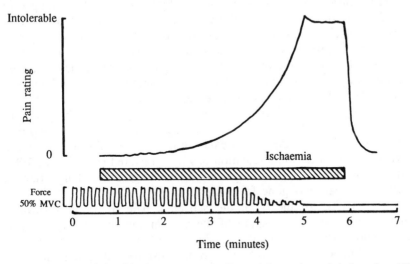

Fig. 10.1 The relationship between contractile activity, pain and ischaemia. The subject performed 50% maximal contractions of the adductor pollicis, first with an intact circulation and then with the circulation occluded. Pain was estimated using an open-ended analogue scale.

Rhythmic submaximal voluntary contractions every one or two

seconds can usually be sustained for long periods without pain, but if the circulation is occluded pain develops (often described as a burning sensation) to reach intolerable levels in a matter of minutes, or less, depending on the force and frequency of the contractions (Fig. 10.1).

When the contractions stop, the pain continues at much the same level until the circulation is restored when it disappears within 10 to 20 seconds. These observations were first made by Sir Thomas Lewis and colleagues in the 1930s who concluded that, as a result of ischaemic exercise, some substance, probably a metabolite, was released from the muscle fibres which, when it accumulated above a certain level, stimulated nociceptors. When the circulation was restored the substance was washed away and the pain resolved. Lewis showed that the onset and intensity of the pain was related to the metabolic cost of the contraction: the higher the force and frequency, the greater the pain developed. Short-term ischaemia by itself does not produce painful sensations but if the muscle is kept without a circulation for 15-30 minutes, appreciable changes in muscle metabolites do occur and the same painful sensations develop.

The identity of the algesic substance remains unknown; potassium, inorganic phosphate and various nucleotides may all be released from fatiguing muscle and could, separately or together, activate pain fibres. The substance could be one of the group which cause vasodilation of capillaries in active muscle. Lactate and hydrogen ions have long been considered to be the cause of all muscle aches and pains but, as with the cause of muscle fatigue (see Chapter 8, Section 8.4.1.2), acidosis cannot be the only cause of pain and is unlikely to be even a major factor. Patients with myophosphorylase deficiency, who cannot produce lactate, rapidly develop pain during ischaemic contractions, and while it is impossible to be certain that the sensations are of the same nature as those felt by normal subjects, the patient's descriptions of the pain, and reactions to it, are the same as those of any normal subject. In addition, in normal subjects, at the end of exercise muscles remains acidic for one or two minutes after the circulation has been restored (Cady *et al*, 1989) and plasma lactate remains high for 10 to 15 minutes, long after the sensation of pain has gone from the muscle.

The motive for the work on ischaemic pain in the 1930s was a desire to understand the nature of the pain in patients with intermittent claudication, where the blood supply to a working limb is compromised. Lewis and his colleagues were able to demonstrate that pathological pain had the same characteristics as pain produced in a normal muscle working under ischaemic conditions. Patients with mitochondrial myopathies or deficiencies of the glycolytic pathway have larger metabolic changes in the muscle for a given amount of exercise and also develop pain in the working muscle more rapidly than normal subjects.

Interestingly, hypothyroid patients, who have a low energy turnover when contracting their muscles, develop muscle pain relatively slowly, emphasising the relationship between metabolic cost and pain during short-term exercise.

10.2.2 *Pain during everyday activities*

Pain is experienced whenever, metabolically, a muscle is failing and no longer in a steady state, that is when the cost of exercise is greater than can be sustained by oxidative metabolism. Running up a flight of steps or carrying heavy loads produce the familiar sensations of pain in the working muscles. The characteristics and, presumably, the causes are the same as for the experimental muscle pain described above, where some algesic substance is thought to be released from the active muscle. The precise level of the algesic substance within the tissue, and hence the level of perceived pain, will be determined by the balance between its production in the tissue and its removal by the perfusing blood. The production and accumulation of lactate in a working muscle is a good example of this mechanism but, as discussed above, lactate cannot be a prime candidate for the algesic substance. Potassium release from working muscles is a more likely cause of the pain. Similarities between the development of pain and the development of fatigue in the working muscle are very striking.

10.3 **Pain developing after exercise**

It is a common experience that heavy or unaccustomed muscular work is associated with a type of pain that becomes evident some hours after the end of exercise and may persist for several days. Discomfort develops in the muscle 6 to 12 hours after the exercise and, typically, a subject will go to bed with only minor discomfort but wake the next morning with severe and, in some cases, almost disabling pain first appreciated while trying to get out of bed. At rest there is little or no discomfort and it is not until the muscle is moved or touched that the pain is experienced. There are a number of sensations of which the two most prominent are stiffness and tenderness, although in severe cases there is also a dull throbbing pain with the muscle at rest.

10.3.1 *Exercise causing delayed onset pain*

Asmussen (1953, 1956) was amongst the first to note that delayed onset pain is caused mainly, if not exclusively, by movements in which the active muscle is stretched, such as whilst walking downhill or lowering weights. This type of movement is often referred to as "eccentric exercise" or "negative work". Muscle groups commonly used to demonstrate this phenomenon are the quadriceps, stretched by stepping down from a box (Newham *et al*, 1983), the calf muscle, exercised by walking backwards down an inclined treadmill (Newham *et al*, 1986), and the elbow flexors, stretched by forcibly extending the forearm (Jones *et al*, 1987a). In every case delayed muscle pain develops only in the muscles which have been stretched. During eccentric contractions large forces are generated in the muscle (see Chapter 2, Section 2.4.4) and tendons but there is none of the burning pain associated with concentric or isometric contractions. Thus, when stepping on and off a high box the leg used to step up, in which the quadriceps muscle shortens and performs work, becomes tired and, if the exercise is fast enough, painful during the test. Any discomfort in this leg is of the type discussed above in Section 10.2 and rapidly resolves. The opposite leg, in which the quadriceps is stretched whilst active and absorbs work lowering the body, is not painful during the exercise. The only unusual sensation is often one of an ill-defined inability to control the muscle, evident as an increasingly heavy landing as the subject steps down. When the elbow flexors are forcibly extended the subject is aware of very high forces in the muscle and tendons but no pain in the muscle. At the end of exercise the subject often has increased tremor in the exercised arm and has difficulty in bending the arm to touch the shoulder. The arm also hangs with the elbow in flexion (Jones *et al*, 1987a).

Although delayed onset muscle pain is most commonly associated with eccentric contractions it can also be induced by high force isometric contractions if the muscle is exercised in an extended position (Jones *et al*, 1989), showing that it is not entirely the high forces that result in muscle pain and that muscle length is an important factor.

10.3.2 *Muscular stiffness*

This sensation is most evident 24 to 48 hours after the exercise when difficulty and pain is experienced stretching the affected muscles, for example when rising from a chair. There is a sensation of mechanical stiffness which gives the feeling that the muscle has become shorter. After eccentric exercise of the elbow flexors there is difficulty straightening the elbow, so that the arm is carried in flexion. If the elbow is straightened forcibly there is a painful stretching sensation in the belly of the muscle. With continuing activity the sensations diminish and after a few minutes of "warm-up" movements become fairly normal but, when the muscle is again rested, the sensations of stiffness return within 10 to 15 minutes with a similar intensity. When stiff, the muscle feels tense and swollen.

Stiffness can be quantified by measuring the force required to forcibly straighten the elbow and is found to be maximal 1 to 2 days after the end of exercise and disappears within about 5 days, a time course that is the same as that of muscle tenderness (Jones *et al*, 1987a).

The stiffness and flexion contracture developed in the exercised forearm flexors is electrically silent, which implies that the muscle fibres are not contracting and that some other structure must be responsible. The most likely explanation is a shortening of the connective tissue arranged in parallel with the muscle fibres (Howell *et al*, 1986; Jones *et al*, 1987a).

10.3.3 *Muscle tenderness*

Tenderness is the unpleasant sensation felt when pressure is applied to a damaged muscle. While at rest or when there is no pressure on the muscle, there is no pain. The degree of tenderness can be measured by recording the threshold pressure required to elicit a painful response (Fig. 10.2). This technique can also be used to map out the painful areas of an exercised muscle (Edwards *et al*, 1981).

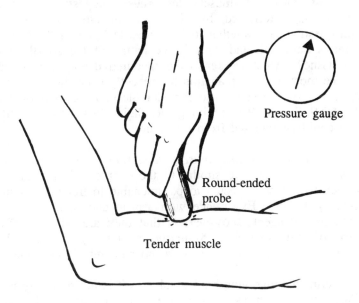

Fig. 10.2 Quantitative assessment of muscle tenderness. A round-ended probe attached to a pressure transducer is pressed into the muscle and the pressure recorded at which pain is first felt.

The feeling is similar to, if not identical with, that around a bruise or tendon sprain. Although it makes many actions unpleasant, for example sitting when the gluteal muscles are affected, there is no indication that tenderness inhibits the activation of muscles during isometric contractions.

After stepping exercise muscle tenderness develops in the quadriceps and gluteal muscles of the leg used to support the body weight whilst stepping down and also in the calf muscle of the contralateral leg. This calf muscle is stretched when the subject touches the ground with a pointed foot and then takes the body weight as the heel comes down to the ground. Eccentric exercise of the elbow flexors produces tenderness in the biceps and brachialis in the upper arm and also the brachioradialis in the lower arm.

The tenderness, which in some cases can make a muscle acutely sensitive to touch, is maximal 1 to 2 days after eccentric exercise and is generally absent or much reduced by 5 days (Fig. 10.3), having a similar time course to the muscle stiffness described above (Section 10.3.2).

10.3.4 *Causes of delayed onset muscle pain*

The slow onset of muscle tenderness suggests a mechanism involving damage followed by some inflammatory process. The important questions are whether it is the muscle fibres or the connective tissue that is damaged, and what is the nature of the signal from the damaged tissue? Most workers have favoured damage to connective tissue as the most likely explanation but recently it has become apparent that eccentric exercise can cause considerable damage to muscle fibres (see Chapter 9, Section 9.3), reviving speculation that the pain-producing substance could be released from this source.

10.3.4.1 *Inflammation and muscle tenderness*   The sensations of tenderness and swelling are similar to those of classical inflammation and as such would be expected to be amenable to treatment with anti-inflammatory agents. Experience with aspirin and other non-steroidal anti-inflammatory agents, however, is that they are without effect on this form of muscle pain. Similarly, a trial of a steroidal anti-inflammatory agent, prednisolone, gave no pain relief (see Jones *et al*, 1987b).

In experiments involving human subjects it is not generally possible to use large doses of drugs or to sample tissues for drug and metabolite levels, so there is always the possibility that the analgesic agent being investigated may not have reached the affected tissue or produced the expected metabolic effect. If muscle tenderness is of the same nature as the tenderness associated with bruising it would be instructive to see whether the pain of a bruise is relieved by aspirin or other anti-inflammatory agents.

10.3.4.2 *Tissue oedema*   Many subjects experiencing muscle tenderness complain of "tightness and swelling" in the affected muscle. Muscles may appear swollen, and increases in circumference of 5 to 10% have been measured. Increased intramuscular pressure is known to give rise to painful sensations in the anterior tibial compartment (splint shins; Matsen, 1979), and tissue oedema, with a consequent rise in pressure, could be a cause of delayed-onset muscle pain in the damaged muscles. Intramuscular pressure has been measured directly in painful and pain-free biceps muscles at intervals after eccentric contractions of the elbow flexors. Resting pressure has been found to be the same in painful and pain-free elbow flexor muscles. Other observations also make it unlikely that increased intramuscular pressure is the immediate cause of muscle tenderness: during isometric contractions of a normal muscle the intramuscular pressure can rise to several hundred mm Hg but this is not perceived as painful in the same way as muscle tenderness and, even in an already tender muscle, isometric contractions do not aggravate the pain.

10.3.4.3 *Release of soluble material from damaged muscle fibres* The release of soluble muscle proteins such as creatine kinase (CK) into the circulation is commonly used as an indication of muscle damage (see Chapter 9).

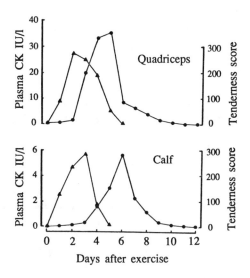

Fig. 10.3 Muscle tenderness and plasma creatine kinase after eccentric exercise of quadriceps and calf muscles. The quadriceps was damaged by 20 minutes stepping and the calf muscles by 2 hours walking backwards down an inclined treadmill. Tenderness (▲); CK (●). CK scale is given × 10³ IU/l.

The time courses of pain development and CK release after eccentric exercise of the calf and quadriceps muscles are shown in Fig. 10.3. The release of CK and development of pain are seen to be clearly dissociated in time and it is therefore unlikely that this particular enzyme is the cause of the pain. CK is a large molecule and it is possible that smaller proteins and peptides could be released at an earlier time when the muscle is painful; a relationship might then still be expected between the extent of muscle damage, as indicated by subsequent CK release, and the severity of the muscle pain. In cases where there is a large CK release there is always considerable pain but the reverse is not always true.

It is notoriously difficult to compare pain scores between subjects, since the reporting of pain is subjective, but there are occasions when it is possible to compare different levels of pain and damage within the same subject. One of the features of eccentric exercise is the rapidity with which the muscle adapts to repeated exercise. Quadriceps tenderness and plasma CK concentration are shown in Fig. 10.4 for a subject who performed a stepping exercise at weekly intervals. During the first week there was a large enzyme release but in the following weeks no significant release occurred.

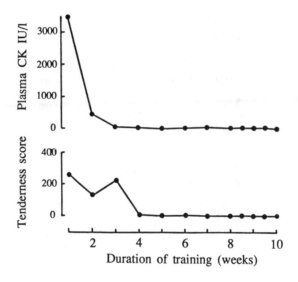

Fig. 10.4 Plasma creatine kinase and quadriceps tenderness with repeated exercise. One subject performed 20 minutes stepping exercise once a week for 10 weeks and the peak values for muscle pain and CK are shown for each week. Note the rapid training effect for plasma CK but a slower reduction in pain.

Although a little reduced, pain was still appreciable during the second and third weeks when there was no evidence of further muscle fibre damage. This demonstrates the poor correlation between tenderness and damage to muscle fibres, suggesting that there is probably no causal relationship.

10.3.4.4 *Reflex activity* On the basis of EMG recordings from painful muscles, De Vries (1966) suggested that damage may result in increased reflex contraction of the muscle and consequent local areas of painful ischaemia. Other studies have produced no evidence to support this view, most investigators finding that painful muscles are electrically silent (Howell *et al*, 1986; Jones *et al*, 1987a). The suggestion also seems unlikely since the acute pain during a contraction (see above, Section 10.2) is not the same sensation as tenderness.

10.3.4.5 *Summary* The immediate cause of delayed onset muscle tenderness remains uncertain but, despite the apparent lack of effect of anti-inflammatory agents, the most likely explanation remains that it is due to an inflammation of the connective tissue in or around the muscle. This inflammation appears to sensitize mechanoreceptors, probably situated in the connective tissue sheaths, so that they respond excessively when the muscle is stretched or pressed.

10.4 The effect of training on muscle pain

Our general experience of life is that, with training, the unpleasant sensation occurring during and after exercise become less evident. The mechanism of the adaptation differs for the two forms of pain. The immediate burning pain associated with high-intensity exercise decreases as a result of training, probably only because the muscle itself develops a better circulation and becomes more resistant to fatigue. For a given level of metabolite depletion it is likely that the pain experienced by a trained and an untrained subject will be the same. There is then another question as to how the two subjects will react to the painful sensation, but that leads into the realms of perception of pain and the psychological adjustments associated with training.

There is no doubt that the sensations of tenderness can be abolished by training (Fig. 10.4). Without knowing the cause of the tenderness it is difficult to specify the changes responsible for the training effect, but it is possible to speculate that, as a result of continued stress on the tendons and muscle fascia, the connective tissue becomes stronger or more elastic, so becoming less susceptible to damage during eccentric exercise. One certain fact is that the training adaptation is specific to the muscle trained. Having trained away the tenderness in one leg the subject illustrated in Fig. 10.4 changed her stepping pattern so that the opposite leg was exercised eccentrically and this leg subsequently developed the characteristic signs of pain and damage.

10.5 Muscle cramp

The pain associated with cramp is distinctive and, in large muscle groups, very distressing. It is associated with major contractions of the affected muscles and the pain may, in part, be similar to the pain developed in a muscle working ischaemically, as discussed above (Section 10.2). This cannot be the complete explanation because cramp pain is felt immediately the contraction begins, as opposed to the 15 to 30-second delay experienced with normal contraction, and the quality is different. There are usually some feelings of discomfort before the muscle goes fully into contraction and afterwards there is a feeling of tenderness not usually associated with even prolonged high-force isometric contractions. Cramps only develop in muscles held in a shortened position and it is sometimes possible to produce cramp-like sensations by voluntarily contracting a muscle in this position.

Cramps are electrically active contractions, unlike the electrically silent contractures, resembling *rigor mortis*, seen in patients with disorders of glycolysis. The process probably involves an increased excitability of the α-motoneurones. Cramps can usually be relieved by stretching the affected muscle, or by stimulation of sensory nerves in the skin, and are possibly prevented by a high sodium intake and quinine, but how effective these treatments are, and how they might work, remains unknown.

10.6 Myalgic pain

Tenderness may develop in muscles, especially in the neck and shoulders, subsequently leading to severe pain, headaches and muscle fixation. This type of pain is experienced by a large proportion of the population and is of considerable economic importance since it affects many people at work carrying out repetitive tasks with their arms. Painful shoulder and neck muscles are also frequently seen following infection with coxsackie B virus. Often areas can be identified from which the pain appears to radiate and these are known as "trigger points". Massage, heat, manipulation and injection of local anaesthetics into these points are often claimed to be of benefit. As with all types of muscle pain, there is speculation that the pain is due to local areas of muscle contraction generating ischaemic pain, possibly as a reflex in response to tissue damage, but evidence for this cause is slight. Biopsies of the trigger points have shown no striking abnormalities and there is no evidence of increased electrical activity in the painful muscle while at rest. The primary lesion could well be in the sensory nerves serving the muscle which, having become sensitized by a viral infection, may transmit inappropriate information.

10.7 References and further reading

Armstrong, R.B. (1984). Mechanisms of exercise induced delayed onset muscular soreness: a brief review. *Medicine and Science in Sports and Exercise* **18**, 529-36.

Asmussen, E. (1953). Positive and negative muscular work. *Acta Physiologica Scandinavia* **28**, 364-82.

Asmussen, E. (1956). Observations on experimental muscle soreness. *Acta Physiologica Scandinavia* **28**, 364-82.

Cady, E.B., Jones, D.A., Lynn, J. & Newham, D.J. (1989). Changes in force and intracellular metabolites during fatigue of human skeletal muscle. *Journal of Physiology* **418**, 311-25.

De Vries, H.A. (1966). Quantitative electromyographic investigation of the spasm theory of muscle pain. *American Journal of Physiological Medicine* **45**, 119-34.

Edwards, R.H.T., Mills, K.R. & Newham, D.J. (1981). Measurement of severity and distribution of experimental muscle tenderness. *Journal of Physiology* **317**, 1-2P.

Howell, J.H., Chila, A.G., Ford, G., David, D. & Gates, T. (1986). An electromyographic study of elbow motion during postexercise muscle soreness. *Journal of applied Physiology* **58**, 1713-18.

Jones, D.A., Newham, D.J. & Clarkson, P.M. (1987a). Skeletal muscle stiffness and pain following eccentric exercise of the elbow flexors. *Pain* **30**, 233-42.

Jones, D.A., Newham, D.J., Obletter, G. & Giamberadino, M.A. (1987b). Nature of exercise-induced muscle pain. In: *Advances in Pain Research and Therapy*, Vol. **10** ed. M. Tengo *et al.* New York, Raven Press, pp. 207-18.

Jones, D.A., Newham, D.J. & Torgan, C. (1989). Mechanical influences on long-lasting human muscle fatigue and delayed onset pain. *Journal of Physiology* **412**, 415-27.

Lewis, T. (1942). *Pain.* New York, Macmillan, esp. pp. 96-104.

Lewis, T., Pickering, G.W. & Rothschild, P. (1931). Observations on muscular pain in intermittent claudication. *Heart* **15**, 359-83.

Matsen, F.A. (1979). Compartmental syndromes. *New England Journal of Medicine* **300**, 1210-11.

Newham, D.J., Jones, D.A. & Edwards, R.H.T. (1986). Plasma creatine kinase after concentric and eccentric contractions. *Muscle and Nerve* **9**, 59-63.

Newham, D.J., Mills, K.R., Quigley, B.M. & Edwards, R.H.T. (1983). Pain and fatigue following concentric and eccentric contractions. *Clinical Science* **64**, 55-62.

Wall, P.D. & Melzack, R.   (ed.), (1989). *Textbook of Pain,*   2nd edition.   London, Churchill Livingstone.

Chapter 11

MUSCLE DISEASES

Muscle diseases present in many different ways. For a child there may be delay in achieving the normal motor milestones such as sitting and walking, an adult may not be able to rise from a chair, climb stairs or turn over in bed, or may experience excessive fatigue. Patients can generally be divided into three groups: (a) those who are weak even when rested; (b) those who are of normal strength at rest but in whom even a small amount of exercise leads to premature or excessive fatigue; and (c) those who are not necessarily weak or especially easily fatigued but have some disturbance of function such as spasticity, inability to relax the muscle after contraction (myotonia), abnormally severe cramps or episodes of weakness. An additional group of patients who are difficult to categorise are those with ill-defined muscle aches and pains. These patients tend to be labelled as hysterical but in many cases this diagnosis merely hides our considerable ignorance of the origins of muscular pain and the perception of fatigue. If any objective evidence of abnormality (in function, structure or chemistry) can be found it is often a great relief to these patients to know that their problem has some organic basis, even if the condition cannot be treated.

The symptom of weakness generally arrises because the patient has lost functional muscle, that is, there has been a loss of contractile material. The primary cause of this loss may be a defect in the muscle itself (myopathy) or in the nervous system innervating that muscle (neuropathy).

The myopathies may be broadly subdivided into two categories; the atrophic myopathies, in which the muscle fibres shrink in size but do not decrease in total number, and the destructive myopathies, where fibres are destroyed and lost. This latter category can be further subdivided into the muscular dystrophies, which are of genetic origin, and the inflammatory myopathies, where the destruction is an autoimmune process. In the neuropathic conditions the muscle fibres become denervated as a result of degeneration of the motor nerve input. This may be as a consequence of degeneration of the motoneurone cell body or of damage to the peripheral axon. In both categories there are disorders which are thought to be of genetic origin and those which are acquired.

Excessive fatiguability is a common complaint, but only in a few cases are there satisfactory explanations for the clinical symptoms. Defects in the glycolytic pathway or the electron transport chain severely limit exercise, but are comparatively rare. Myasthenia gravis, an autoimmune disorder, affects the post-synaptic membrane of the neuromuscular junction and leads to a rapid loss of force during sustained efforts.

Abnormalities of muscle function are also relatively rare but are of great interest from the physiological standpoint as they provide ways of understanding cellular mechanisms. Most are associated with changes in the electrical properties of the muscle fibre membrane which render the fibre either over- or under-excitable.

The following chapter can only give an outline of the major disease catagories affecting skeletal muscle and the interested reader is referred to larger specialist works for more detail. The general histochemical appearance and muscle pathology are well illustrated by Anderson (1985). Dubowitz (1985) deals with the atrophic myopathies and the dystrophies, while Walton (1981) covers the neuropathies. Inflammatory disorders of muscle are discussed by Morrow and Isenberg (1987) and Edwards and Jones (1983) provide a summary of the disorders affecting fatiguability and of those giving rise to changes in excitability of the muscle.

A brief summary of muscle disorders is provided at the end of this chapter (Section 11.13).

11.1 Atrophic myopathies

Atrophic myopathies are some of the most commonly encountered causes of weakness and muscle wasting and they are frequently secondary to a clinical condition affecting some other system. The muscle wasting is due to a reduction in the cross-sectional area of individual muscle fibres, often affecting one fibre type more than another. Most frequently it is the type 2 fibres that show the greatest atrophy (Fig. 11.1). Type 2 fibre atrophy is commonly seen in hypothyroidism, osteomalacia, Cushing's syndrome, chronic alcoholism, prolonged steroid therapy and in the wasting which occurs as a result of malignant disease or malnutrition. It is not known why the fast type 2 fibres are more often affected. One theory is that they atrophy as a result of the inactivity caused by the primary clinical problem, but limited studies on patients with atrophy after limb immobilisation suggest that in this situation it is the type 1 fibres which are more severely affected. Alternatively, it is possible that the type 2 fibres represent a pool of protein which is utilised by the body during times of stress, fast fibres being less essential for survival than the fatigue-resistant type 1 fibres.

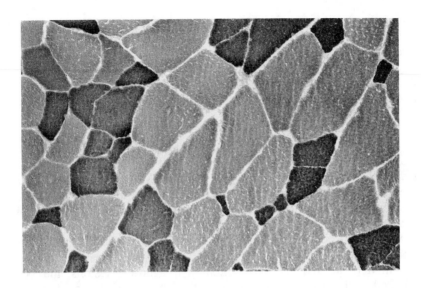

Fig. 11.1 Type 2 fibre atrophy. There is a reduction in the size of the type 2 (dark) fibres; ATPase pH 9.4.

Preferential atrophy of type 1 fibres is less common; it has been reported in myotonic dystrophy, in some childhood myopathies and, as mentioned above, in the quadriceps muscles of patients who have been immobilised for some time after knee injury or lower limb fracture. A complete absence of type 1 fibres can be seen in biopsies from the quadriceps of paraplegic patients after traumatic transection of the spinal cord.

In most cases of atrophic myopathy, if the underlying disorder can be successfully treated, muscle strength and size usually recover, with the atrophic fibres growing back to their full size, although this can be a slow process taking many months.

11.2 Inflammatory myopathies

Polymyositis and dermatomyositis are the most commonly seen types of inflammatory myopathy. Most authorities consider them to be variants of the same disorder which has an incidence of 0.5 per 100,000 and a prevalence of 8 per 100,000. Both diseases are almost certainly the result of autoimmune processes with a female to male preponderance of about 3:1. Inflammatory myopathies have been classified by Bohan and Peters (1975) under the following headings:

Group 1:   Primary idiopathic polymyositis.
Group 2:   Primary idiopathic adult dermatomyositis.
Group 3:   Dermatomyositis with polymyositis associated with neoplasia.
Group 4:   Childhood dermatomyositis associated with vasculitis.
Group 5:   Polymyositis or dermatomyositis associated with collagen vascular disease.

The inflammatory changes lead to a loss of muscle tissue, weakness, gradual immobilisation of the patient and, if the respiratory muscles are involved, may result in respiratory failure. Muscle tenderness is often present, the plasma creatine kinase (CK) may be markedly elevated and a myopathic EMG is often, but not always, found. Cardiac abnormalities have been reported and myoglobinuria due to the release of soluble protein from the damaged muscles may, in severe cases, lead to renal failure.

In dermatomyositis, in addition to the muscle lesions, the skin is affected with lilac discolouration of the upper eyelids and face and a patchy erythematous rash over the hands and sometimes the forearms.

The main pathological changes seen in a muscle biopsy are muscle fibre degeneration and necrosis with inflammatory infiltration in perivascular, perimysial and endomysial areas (Fig. 11.2a & b). Atrophied fibres, particularly in perifasicular areas, and fibres with abnormal architecture may be seen. Regenerating fibres are often present in acute cases but are less often seen in chronic polymyositis, where degenerate fibres are replaced by fat and fibrous tissue (Fig. 11.2c).

Treatment is with steroids and other anti-inflammatory agents, but careful monitoring of the steroid therapy is necessary to maximise effects on the immune system while minimising the tendency of corticosteroids to put the patient into negative nitrogen balance leading to further loss of strength due to fibre atrophy, particularly of the type 2 fibres.

The appearance of biopsies from patients with inflammatory disorders of muscle are shown in Fig. 11.2. As has been discussed in Chapter 9 (Section 9.3) and illustrated in Fig. 9.7, there are many similarities between the appearance of the pathological specimens and that of normal muscle which has been experimentally damaged. This observation suggests that the cellular infiltration seen in polymyositis and dermatomyositis may be part of a normal response to abnormal or damaged muscle, thus pointing to a change in the muscle rather than a defective immune system.

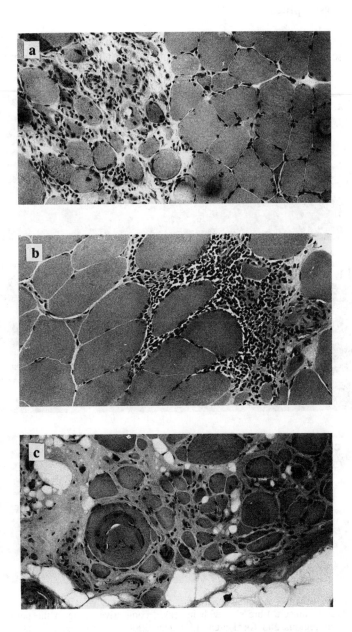

Fig. 11.2 Inflammatory myopathy. Biopsy samples from quadriceps muscles. **a**, the
fascicle on the left shows a typical inflammatory infiltrate. **b**, perimysial inflammatory
infiltrate. **c**, advanced polymyositis. Fat and fibrous tissue have replaced contractile
tissue and bizarre fibre forms are seen. All haematoxylin and eosin stain.

11.3 **Dystrophies**

The term *muscular dystrophy* includes all hereditary progressive disorders
of muscle which result in fibre destruction and the relentless replacement
of muscle cells with fat and fibrous tissue.

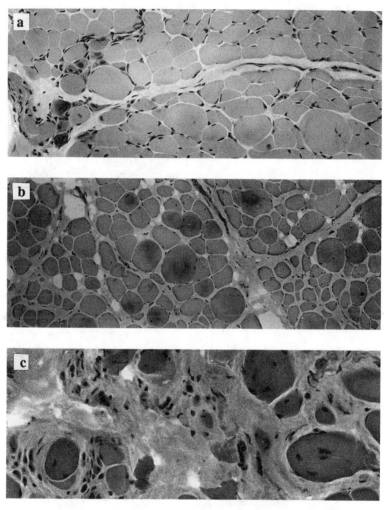

Fig. 11.3 Duchenne muscular dystrophy. **a**, boy aged 2 yrs, quadriceps muscle; note
differences in muscle fibre size with increased connective tissue in the perimysial and
endomysial regions and focal areas of regeneration. **b**, boy aged 9 yrs, quadriceps;
there is fibre hypertrophy and atrophy, some fibres have internal nuclei, note the
marked proliferation of connective tissue. **c**, boy aged 18 yrs, gastrocnemius muscle;
the few remaining fibres are surrounded by fat and connective tissue. Haematoxylin
and eosin stains.

In most dystrophies light microscopy reveals wide variations in fibre size and a tendency to internalisation of the normally subsarcolemmal nuclei (Fig. 11.3a & b), some increase in cellularity, and increased lysosomal activity which can be seen in fibres stained for acid phosphatase. In addition, numerous large, round hyaline fibres and small basophilic fibres are seen; the latter are thought to be regenerating cells. As the condition progresses the increase in fat and connective tissue becomes more marked until virtually no contractile material remains (Fig. 11.3c).

The most serious, though not the most common, type is *Duchenne muscular dystrophy* (DMD). Incidence figures for this disease vary from 13 to 33 per 100,000 live male births with a prevalence in the population of 1.9 to 3.4 per 100,000. It has a sex linked recessive mode of inheritance so that boys are affected but girls act as carriers.

If there is no family history the condition may not be noticed at first as there are few physical signs of the disease at birth (although plasma CK can be as high as 10,000 IU/l), but by 3 to 4 years a delay in reaching the usual motor milestones becomes apparent. Subsequently the child has increasing difficulty standing and walking and by the beginning of the second decade is usually confined to a wheelchair. As the disease progresses, weakness of the respiratory muscles, often accentuated by scolliosis, becomes a problem and death usually occurs before the third decade. Life expectancy depends on the quality of nursing care available, major aims being to minimise contractures and to prevent the development of the respiratory problems which lead to congestion, infections and often a fatal pneumonia.

The defective gene in DMD has now been assigned to a deletion in position Xp21 on the short arm of the X chromosome. The gene is large, spanning a genomic region of about 2,000 kb, and the protein encoded for by this region has been identified and named *dystrophin*. Monoclonal antibodies raised against dystrophin have shown its location to be at the periphery of muscle fibres in association with the plasma membrane and it is thought to have a structural role in the surface membrane. Isolation of DNA segments from the Xp21 region has provided probes which are useful for the prenatal diagnosis of DMD in mothers known to be at risk. Nevertheless, even with the most efficient prenatal screening the incidence of DMD will still remain significant, because spontaneous mutations in this large gene are responsible for about one-third of all reported cases.

The clinically less severe form, *Becker muscular dystrophy*, is now known to be allelic with the more severe disease, with an incidence said to be one-tenth to one-fifth and the prevalence one-third to one-half that of the Duchenne form. In Becker dystrophy the production of dystrophin appears to be reduced and variable in amount. The essential pathological features are the same and the course is progressive in both forms but with a slower time course in Becker dystrophy, where patients may survive into the fourth or fith decades.

Fascioscapulohumeral dystrophy is another well-recognised form of muscular dystrophy. Inheritance is dominant but there is a wide variety of gene expression within families. Patients usually have a normal life span. Distribution of weakness is predominantly in the upper limb-girdle but later in the disease the lower limbs may also be affected. Also dominantly inherited is *Occulopharyngeal dystrophy* in which abnormalities of mitochondrial structure and function and changes of immune tolerance have been reported. Other forms of dystrophy include the X-linked recessive *Emery-Dreifuss humeroperoneal* form, the autosomal recessive and relatively benign *limb girdle dystrophy* and the *scapulohumeral* form which also has an autosomal recessive inheritance and is characterised by cardiomyopathy and contractures. An absence of dystrophin does not appear to be associated with any of these dystrophies.

In clinical practice the most likely form of dystrophy to be encountered in adults is *myotonic dystrophy*. This is dominantly inherited with variable gene penetration, and the gene maps on chromosome 19 in the q13.2-13.3 region. Incidence is calculated to be 13.5 per 100,000. Weakness starts peripherally and only later are proximal muscle groups involved. Myotonia of the hands is often the initial symptom. This is a multi-system disease in which many organs, including brain, heart, endocrine organs, skin and eyes are affected. Although giving its name to the disorder, myotonia itself is not the major problem.

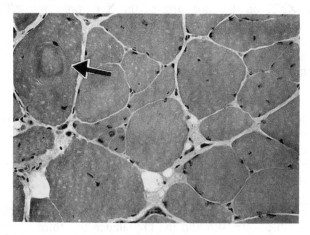

Fig. 11.4   Myotonic dystrophy, quadriceps muscle from a girl age 17 yrs; note differences in fibre size, some fibres showing marked hypertrophy, one bizarre fibre (arrow), numerous internal nuclei and some proliferation of connective tissue. H&E.

Light microscopy of skeletal muscle biopsies reveals differences in fibre size, the type 1 fibres frequently being smaller than the type 2 fibres. Numerous internal nuclei and, in longitudinal sections, nuclear chains are also seen. As the disease progresses, variability in the size of both fibre types becomes more extreme and is accompanied by architectural changes in the fibres, with a generalised increase in fibrosis.

Among the disorders of muscle which occur *in utero* are the autosomal recessive *congenital muscular dystrophies* in which the infants are born with weakness and hypotonia and a "dystrophic" muscle biopsy picture. The disease, however, progresses little after birth.

11.4 Congenital myopathies

Congenital myopathies may manifest as a failure in the development of one particular fibre type leading to a predominance of the other (usually type 1), or the presence within the muscle fibres of rod-like bodies (*nemeline myopathy*) or cores (*central core disease*). These are disorders of early childhood which remain static or progress slowly.

11.5 Neuropathies

Muscle requires an intact, healthy and active nerve supply for its development and normal function and damage to the nervous supply leads to pathological changes in the muscle. Three groups of neurogenic muscle disease can be identified according to the site of the lesion: (1) lesions in the anterior horn cells, as in the *spinal muscular atrophies* and *motor neurone disease*; (2) axonal lesions, as in *peripheral neuropathies*; and (3) lesions at the motor end plate as in *myasthenia gravis*.

11.5.1 *Muscle biopsy appearance*

The microscopic appearance of a muscle biopsy specimen can give important information about the differential diagnosis and the progress of the disorder. There are a number of features of a muscle biopsy that, if present, immediately suggest a neuropathic cause.

The muscle fibres constituting a single motor unit are widely distributed throughout the muscle so that loss of a motoneurone or damage to an axon or its peripheral branches will result in the appearance of scattered atrophic muscle fibres (often referred to as *small angular fibres*), also widely distributed throughout the muscle (Fig. 11.5a). As increasing numbers of motoneurones are affected so the chances increase of adjacent muscle fibres becoming atrophied, which leads to clumps of small fibres and is known as *small group atrophy* (Fig. 11.5b). Since adjacent fibres will probably be supplied by different motoneurones, atrophy of neuropathic origin is of both fibre types and so can be distinguished from the muscle fibre atrophy described in Section 11.1, which is usually predominantly of one fibre type.

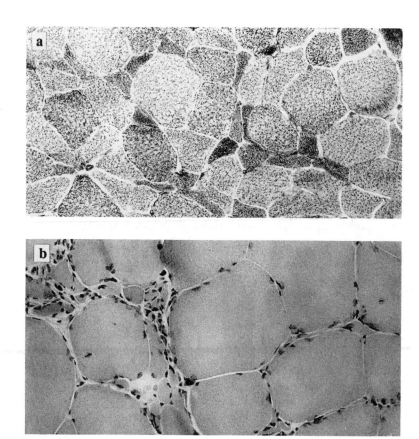

Fig. 11.5 **a**, scattered small angular fibres due to denervation. Quadriceps muscle, NADH-TR stain. **b**, motor neurone disease; small group atrophy, a group of atrophic denervated fibres are seen between normal fibre forms. H&E stain.

Another neuropathic feature is known as *large group atrophy* in which large areas of atrophic fibres, often whole fascicles, are seen which involve both fibre types (Fig. 11.6a). It is possible that large group atrophy may occur by coincidence, in that all the motoneurones supplying one fascicle happen to have failed, but this seems a little unlikely. Alternatively, it is possible that the defect might originate in the fascicle itself. This is of particular interest in relation to the aetiology of motor neurone disease (see below).

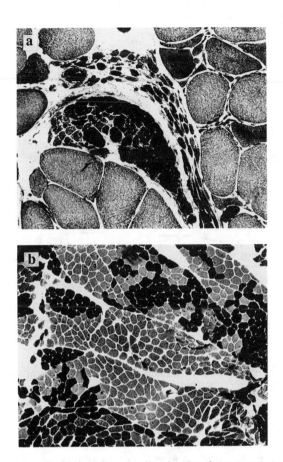

Fig. 11.6 **a**, chronic spinal muscular atrophy showing large group atrophy: whole fascicles are affected. NADH-TR stain. **b**, fibre type grouping, quadriceps muscle, woman aged 42 yrs. Groups of one fibre type denote reinnervation. ATPase pH 9.4.

If the condition becomes chronic, evidence of reinnervation appears, leading to fibre type grouping. Mature muscle fibres are innervated by a single axon, but if the innervation is lost, nearby undamaged axons sprout and branch to form new contacts with the denervated muscle fibre. Initially there may be multiple innervation, which undergoes the same process of selection and elimination as seen in foetal muscle (Chapter 3). If the process of denervation and reinnervation occurs and reoccurs over a long period, one healthy axon comes to dominate an area of muscle and all the fibres assume the contractile and histochemical characteristics set by its motorneurone. This change is seen in muscle biopsy sections as groups of muscle fibres which are all of the same fibre type in contrast to the random arrangement of fibre types seen in healthy muscle (Fig. 11.6b).

As the muscle fibres of one motor unit are grouped together, synchronous action potentials will be recorded, giving rise to the characteristic "giant action potentials" seen on EMG examination (Fig. 11.7).

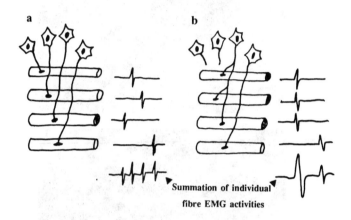

Fig. 11.7 **a**, normal muscle with fibres innervated by different motoneurones. The activity recorded is the summation of asynchronous activity in the fibres. **b**, muscle after denervation and re-innervation. A single motoneurone supplies a group of fibres giving a *giant* action potential.

11.5.2 *Disorders of the lower motoneurone*

There are a large number of disorders which result in the degeneration of motoneurones. Broadly they may be divided into those disorders where the degeneration appears to have a genetic cause, for instance the *spinal muscular atrophies*, and those where the disease is acquired (or at least thought to be so) as a result of infection or contact with a toxic substance. The latter include *motor neurone diseases* and *poliomyelitis*.

11.5.2.1 *Motor neurone disease (amyotrophic lateral sclerosis)* This is a disease of middle to old age, with a male predominance, and is characterised by widespread degeneration of motoneurones. Although familial forms exist the majority of cases are sporadic and of late onset. The disease has a worldwide distribution and is responsible for 1 in 1000 adult deaths, and there is an annual incidence of approximately 1 to 2 per 100,000 population and a prevalence of 2.5 per 100,000.

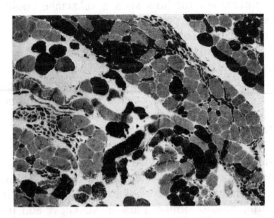

Fig. 11.8   Motor neurone disease. Groups of atrophied fibres are of both fibre types. ATPase pH 9.4.

The first clinical signs often appear in the distal small muscles of the hand and in most cases the disease progresses rapidly to a global weakness. The combination of upper and lower motoneurone lesions is characterised by wasting and fasciculation of the limb muscles with spasticity and brisk reflexes. The duration from clinical onset to death rarely exceeds 3 years.

The disease is unusually common in three distinct geographical locations, the Pacific island of Guam, the Kiwi peninsula of Japan and New Guinea, and this has lead to speculation about the involvement of specific environmental factors including the toxic effects of manganese, aluminium and lead. The introduction of American dietary habits to these areas has been associated with a reduction in the incidence of the disease and it is possible that a high calcium intake may protect against aluminium poisoning.   Neurotropic viruses have been sought, unsuccessfully, and an autoimmune component has been suggested.

The central nervous system is generally well protected by the blood-brain barrier but motoneurones have extensive terminations in muscle where they are not protected in this way. It is well established that there is transport of macromolecules both down and up the axon and retrograde transport of toxins has been demonstrated from the periphery to the cell body. If, in the case illustrated in Figs. 11.6 and 11.8, there had been some toxin in the atrophic fascicles, it could have been transported back to kill all the motoneurones innervating fibres in that fascicle. This would lead to the microscopic pattern often seen, namely group atrophy at the site where the toxin originated and a diffuse distribution of small angular fibres in the rest of the muscle. There are obvious difficulties with this theory; there is no known candidate for the toxin and no explanation for how such a substance could originate and remain localised in a small portion of muscle.

Another explanation for motoneurone disease is that motoneurones require continual stimulation by trophic substances secreted by the muscle and carried along the motor axon back to the cell body. It is suggested that failure of this process leads to death of the motoneurone. This is seen as analogous to the extensive loss of motoneurones which occurs in the foetus when superfluous axonal terminations are eliminated from the maturing muscle fibres.

11.5.2.2 *Poliomyelitis*   In this virus infection there is destruction and necrosis of the anterior horn cells leading to profound muscle weakness. Other viruses, for example the coxsackie viruses, can also invade anterior horn cells, giving rise to similar muscle weakness and paralysis. This disease is similar to the condition of *distemper* in dogs.

11.5.2.3   *Proximal spinal muscular atrophy (hereditary motor neuropathy)*   The spinal muscular atrophies are a group of genetic disorders characterised by degeneration of anterior horn cells, the motor nuclei in the brain stem and, rarely, the upper motoneurone pathways. The genetic defect is unknown and the various types are distinguished by the age of onset and the distribution of weakness. In recent years the view that several separate genes are involved has been strengthened by large family studies. The main forms are:

1.   *Acute infantile (SMA type 1: Werdnig-Hoffman disease)*, autosomal recessive (AR) inheritance. This disorder is characterised by its severe generalised muscle involvement and fatal outcome within the first 2 years of life. It is thought to be due to a single autosomal recessive gene. There is an estimated disease incidence of 1 per 20,000 live births. In about one-third of cases the disease becomes evident before birth with decreased foetal movements. It is one of the many causes of a floppy infant but gross weakness and global paresis create a distinctive clinical picture. There is evidence of delayed motor milestones by 6 months of age and feeding difficulties and breathing problems are common. Cardiac muscle is not affected.

2.   *Chronic childhood (SMA type II, Arrested Werdnig-Hoffman disease)*, AR inheritance. This is a milder juvenile form; a single autosomal recessive gene is thought to account for 90% of these cases.

3.   *Adult onset chronic proximal (SMA type III: Kugelberg-Welander disease)*, AR inheritance. This is not a variant of the childhood form. It is a relatively benign condition and life span is usually normal.

4. *Chronic proximal juvenile onset (SMA type IV)*, autosomal dominant (AD) inheritance. This is the mildest form. Onset is late and the children are able to walk and generally remain mobile for many years. The clinical picture is very similar to a limb-girdle muscular dystrophy. Many patients in this group have a normal life span.

5. *Adult onset (SMA type V)*, AD inheritance. This is very similar to SMA type III but with a dominant inheritance. Rare X-linked forms have been described.

Other forms of SMA occur which predominantly affect either the distal muscles or cause scapuloperineal or facioscapulohumeral distributions of weakness. Varied inheritance patterns, both AR and AD, occur in these groups.

11.5.2.4 *Muscle biopsy in SMA* It is not possible to distinguish between acute and chronic infantile SMA by muscle biopsy as the appearances are identical. There is severe grouped atrophy, and sometimes whole fascicles are composed of tiny rounded fibres which the ATPase reaction shows to be of both fibre types with a normal checker-board distribution. In other fascicles, groups of normal fibres and others of grossly hypertrophied fibres (Fig. 11.9) are seen, the latter often being of one fibre type (usually type 1).

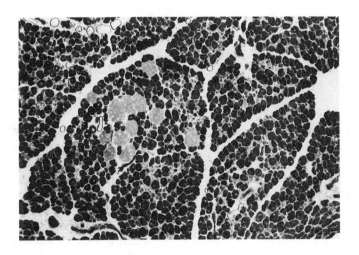

Fig 11.9 Acute infantile SMA. A group of grossly hypertrophied type 1 fibres is seen centre field. ATPase pH 9.4.

In chronic proximal and other milder forms of SMA, group atrophy with small clusters of atrophic fibres is seen. Pyknotic nuclear clusters may occur and there may be evidence of reinnervation with fibre type grouping. Very large fibres are not a feature. Target and whorled fibres and other architectural fibre abnormalities are common. In more advanced cases replacement of fibres by fat and fibrous tissue may occur.

11.5.3 *Peripheral neuropathies*

Peripheral neuropathies are diseases characterised by structural damage and functional loss in the peripheral nervous system which can be due to physical damage, inflammatory disease, metabolic factors (e.g. diabetes), toxic factors (e.g. alcohol abuse or poisoning with heavy metals), or may be genetic in origin. The incidence of peripheral nerve disease is probably higher than that of primary muscle disease. Impairment of both sensory and motor function can occur, although one or the other may dominate the clinical picture. Only those diseases with a significant motor nerve component will result in muscle weakness. The peripheral nerve pathology may be segmental demyelination or axonal degeneration. In demyelinating neuropathies there is usually a marked slowing of nerve conduction which is not seen in axonal degeneration, providing that some large fast conducting axons remain. Distal segments of the limbs are usually most severely affected. There is a vast pathological spectrum and two of the commonest are discussed below.

11.5.3.1 *Hereditary motor and sensory neuropathy (HMSN)* In this syndrome a convenient classification is by the velocity of peripheral nerve conduction. In *HMSN Type I* a low conduction velocity is associated with segmental demyelination and hypertrophy of the nerves that can be palpated (onion bulb). This is a result of Schwann cell proliferation accompanying remyelination. Onset is usually within the first 10 years of life. Normal conduction velocity is seen in *HMSN type II* in which there is axonal degeneration and only minimal demyelination. Onset after 40 years of age is quite common in this form which may be associated with upper motoneurone lesions or the clinical picture of Friedreich's ataxia. Patients may develop *inverted champagne bottle* or *stork* legs (fat thighs, thin calves).

Muscle biopsy of the lower limb muscles in the early stages of the disease shows mild denervation atrophy which resembles the less severe demyelinating disorder. Later, in the type II form, small group atrophy with muscle fibre type grouping reflects the occurrence of reinnervation. There may be compensatory hypertrophy of the remaining fibres.

11.5.3.2 *Acute acquired peripheral neuropathy* The *Guillain-Barré syndrome* of acute post-infective polyneuropathy is probably the commonest acquired peripheral neuropathy associated with muscle weakness. Typically, an acute febrile illness is followed by generalised weakness of both proximal and distal muscles which may become so severe that assisted ventilation is required. The condition is due to inflammatory segmental demyelination which appears on nerve conduction examination as a slowing or complete block of nerve conduction. Severe demyelination may produce secondary axonal degeneration. In most cases remyelination occurs and the patient recovers, but some cases may be left with residual weakness. Relapses occasionally occur.

Changes seen in the muscle biopsy depend on the severity of the axonal degeneration, where this is severe small group atrophy is seen.

11.6 Diseases of the neuromuscular junction

11.6.1 *Myasthenia gravis*

Myasthenia gravis is a disease characterised by the development of weakness and abnormal fatigue. After a period of inactivity the muscles recover normal strength but weakness develops again after only brief activity. All muscles of the body may be involved but weakness of the facial muscles with drooping eyelids often gives the patient a characteristic appearance. There may be difficulty with speech and swallowing and involvement of the respiratory muscles can prove fatal. Onset can be at any age and may be rapid or insidious, but it is most common in the third and fourth decades of life. The incidence is between 1 per 10,000 and 1 per 50,000 of the population, with twice as many females as males affected.

Diagnostic features are the characteristic EMG picture and an often dramatic improvement in muscle strength after injection of the cholinesterase inhibitor *edrophonium chloride* (the "Tensilon test"). Another test may be used in which the response of the muscle to brief stimulation at 3 Hz is measured. In myasthenia a decrement in action potential size is seen. During sustained activity there is a reduction in the quantal release of acetylcholine. With normal muscle this is of little consequence as there is a large margin of safety but in myasthenia the natural transmitter is competing with a curare-like inhibitor. In this situation a fall in transmitter release causes the number of miniature end plate potentials (MEPPs) generated to fall below the threshold required to initiate a propagated action potential in the muscle fibre.

Normal nerve conduction velocities and the beneficial effects of cholinesterase inhibitors show that the site of the lesion in myasthenia is at the neuromuscular junction. The disease is an autoimmune process in which circulating antibodies can be demonstrated. These have two actions: the first is a curare-like inhibition of the neuromuscular junction, the second is an effect on the turnover of acetyl choline receptors, giving rise to abnormally flattened post-synaptic membranes with few junctional folds.

Thymectomy is often helpful if carried out early in the disease but later, when antibody production is at extrathymic sites, thymectomy is ineffective. Plasmapheresis to remove circulating antibody can give temporary relief but long-term management of the autoimmune condition is usually with steroids or immunosuppressive drugs. Anticholinesterase inhibitors effectively relieve the myasthenic symptoms and it is important to find a preparation which will give relief during periods of activity but will not have toxic side-effects.

11.6.2 *The Lambert Eaton myasthenic syndrome*

The Lambert Eaton syndrome is, like myasthenia gravis, a condition characterised by weakness and fatigue, and may also be associated with abnormalities of the autonomic nervous system. The disease is more common in men and can present at any age but in the older age groups it is often associated with malignancy, particularly small-cell carcinoma of the lung. EMG findings indicate the presence of a block in neurotransmission which improves with continuing activity. The defect, which, unlike the case of myasthenia gravis, is in the presynaptic membrane, appears to be due to an autoimmune process, antibodies being produced against the active zone particles of the presynaptic cleft from which acetylcholine is released. The condition responds well to corticosteroid therapy (Engel, 1987).

11.7 Neuromuscular changes in human immunodeficiency virus (HIV) infection

During the past few years reports have appeared of neuromuscular diseases associated with HIV infections. These include *Guillain-Barré syndrome* and other peripheral neuropathies, type 2 fibre atrophy, a necrotising myopathy and a polymyositis-like syndrome with a raised creatine kinase and a myopathic EMG. Electron microscopic examination of muscle biopsies has also revealed mitochondrial abnormalities.

Some myopathic changes are thought to be related to use of the drug Zidovudine (AZT), which is used in the treatment of HIV-positive individuals to protect against the development of AIDS-related complex. The type of neuropathy or myopathy encountered seems to be related to the specific stage of HIV infection and chronic asymptomatic HIV infection should be considered, particularly in high-risk individuals, in the differential diagnosis of certain acquired polyneuopathies and muscle disorders.

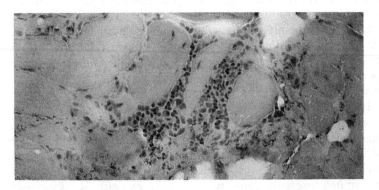

Fig. 11.10 Inflammatory infiltrate in the quadriceps muscle of an HIV positive man aged 42 years who was being treated with AZT. Haematoxylin and eosin.

11.8 Post-viral fatigue syndrome (myalgic encephalomyelitis)

Patients with this syndrome present with an array of symptoms but one of the main complaints is of excessive fatigue after mild exercise; delayed onset muscle pain may also occur. Psychological problems, particularly depression, are also a common feature. Persistence of virus particles from an original precipitating infection, abnormal muscle membrane conductance, excessive intracellular acidosis during exercise and disturbance of the T4 to T8 lymphocyte ratio have all been reported. Opinions differ, sometimes sharply, as to whether the problem is a psychological disorder or one in which there is an abnormality of skeletal muscle function. Tests of muscle function are usually inconclusive or normal but this may reflect the difficulty of devising tests that truly reflect the activity of daily life. Muscle biopsy in these cases generally show only non-specific changes with rather small mean fibre areas and low oxidative capacity which might simply reflect under use of the muscles. The condition covers a wide variety of problems and overlaps with a similar set of symptoms, known as *effort syndrome*. The fact that the symptoms are generally similar to those of any healthy person who is very tired as a result of excess mental or physical effort raises the possibility that the patients may have a heightened awareness of the normal aches and pains of everyday life (see Chapter 8 for a discussion of the sensations associated with fatigue).

11.9 Disorders of energy metabolism

There are a number of rare genetically-determined conditions which give rise to defects in muscle energy metabolism. These include defects in the enzymes of the glycolytic pathway, mitochondrial enzymes concerned with both pyruvate and fatty acid metabolism, and the cytochrome components of the electron transport chain. All of these pathways are important in the secondary supply of energy to muscles as the primary reserve of phosphocreatine becomes depleted.

In general, patients with metabolic defects are of normal or near-normal strength when rested but are limited in their exercise endurance. When a defect occurs in the glycolytic pathway the exercised muscle tends to go into a painful contracture (an electrically silent contraction similar to rigor mortis). Patients with mitochondrial disorders have a very limited exercise capacity and mild exercise is associated with breathlessness, acidosis and high blood lactate as would be seen with a normal muscle exercising under hypoxic conditions.

11.9.1 *Glycolytic disorders*

Research into metabolic disorders of skeletal muscle began with the discovery in 1951 of a myopathy where there was a defect in glycolysis (*McArdle's disease*). In this disease there is a specific lack of the adult form of *myophosphorylase*, the first enzyme in the pathway utilising muscle glycogen.

Patients have normal strength at rest but pain is experienced in the muscles during exercise which becomes severe if exercise is continued at the same intensity. There is rapid fatigue, and the muscle may go into a painful contracture. A period of rest or more gentle exercise often leads to diminution of the pain (the *second wind* phenomenon) and the ability to continue exercise for a time. The absence of myophosphorylase means that the muscle is unable to utilise stored glycogen which severely limits its ability to function under anaerobic conditions. The second wind phenomenon is a result of the utilisation of blood-borne substrates such as glucose and fatty acids by the muscle as an alternative to muscle glycogen. Patients can be helped by eating carbohydrates to raise blood glucose just before exercise. The specific enzyme defect can be demonstrated histochemically in sections from a muscle biopsy specimen: large amounts of glycogen are also seen in the muscle fibres of patients with McArdle's disease.

McArdle's disease is now categorised as type 5 in a group of glycogenoses. A summary of these conditions is given below.

Type 1. *Von Gierke's disease.* Here there is a deficiency of the enzyme *glucose-6-phosphatase* leading to hepatomegaly, growth retardation, hypoglycaemia and lactic acidosis. The liver, kidney and skeletal muscles are affected.

Type 2. *Pompe's disease (acid maltase deficiency).* The lysosomal enzymes α-*1,4* and α-*1,6 glucosidase* are deficient. In children all tissues are affected with a cardiomyopathy and severe weakness with large accumulations of glycogen in the muscle. Death is usually within the first year of life. In adults the disease may present with a proximal myopathy of variable severity and weakness of the respiratory muscles.

Type 3. *Cori-Forbes disease (debrancher deficiency).* The absence of debrancher enzyme leads to the production of limit dextrin as the myophosphorylase enzyme removes from glycogen the glycosyl units attached by 1,4 linkages but cannot attack any branch points. This abnormal glycogen accumulates in the muscle. Clinical symptoms vary from severe muscle weakness in childhood to asymptomatic adult forms.

Type 4. *Andersen's disease (brancher deficiency).* The absence of brancher enzyme results in the deposition of large amounts of abnormal glycogen in childhood. The disease is rapidly progressive, with cirrhosis and hepatosplenomegaly.

Type 5. *McArdle's disease.* In this condition the enzyme myophosphorylase is deficient. The disease is discussed above.

Type 6. *Her's disease.* The liver enzyme *glycogen phosphorylase* is deficient, leading to hepatomegaly, hypoglycaemia and lactic acidosis. The skeletal muscles are not affected.

Type 7. *Tauri's disease.* Here the enzyme *phosphofructokinase* is deficient in skeletal muscle and red cells. The clinical symptoms and exercise impairment are very similar to those of McArdle's disease. Because the deficiency is also present in the red cells a haemolytic anaemia may occur, often detectable by a raised reticulocyte count in the peripheral blood.

11.9.2 Mitochondrial defects

Microscopic examination of muscle from patients with mitochondrial myopathies shows characteristic *ragged red* fibres (Fig. 11.11). This abnormal staining is due to subsarcolemmal aggregations of defective mitochondria. Mitochondrial myopathies are associated with profound exercise intolerance in adults and muscle weakness and hypotonia in babies and young children.

A variety of defects including the transport of pyruvate into mitochondria, lack of pyruvate dehydrogenase and defects in the electron transport chain have been described, all of which will reduce oxidative metabolism. The inheritance of mitochondrial disorders is unique since the mitochondrial DNA, which codes for 13 protein components of the electron transport chain, is transmitted exclusively by the mother (Harding, 1989). Poor oxidative metabolism has two consequences, a reduction in the rate of ATP synthesis and an accumulation of lactate and pyruvate leading to metabolic acidosis. Even with an intact circulation the muscles in these patients are continually working under effectively hypoxic conditions and their muscle function is like that of a normal subject working ischaemically.

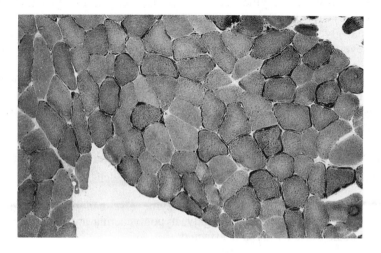

Fig. 11.11 Mitochondrial myopathy. Dark staining at the periphery of the fibres caused by aggregation of mitochondria. TS quadriceps muscle, trichrome stain.

11.9.3 *Disorders of fat metabolism*

Disorders of fat metabolism should properly be classified under mitochondrial myopathies, but because defects in fatty acid metabolism do not have such a drastic effect on energy supply as defects in the electron transport chain, they are considered separately. Patients with disorders of fatty acid metabolism have symptoms of weakness, exercise intolerance, muscle stiffness and pain (sometimes accompanied by myoglobinuria). Symptoms are most evident at times when free fatty acids are the main substrates for energy metabolism, such as during prolonged submaximal exercise, particularly in the fasting state. The β-oxidation of fatty acids depends on the transport of free fatty acids into the mitochondria by a shuttle mechanism involving carnitine and the carnitine palmitoyltransferase (CPT) enzymes. Low plasma and muscle carnitine and deficiencies of CPT have been described. Patients lacking in carnitine are weak whereas those lacking CPT enzymes are of fairly normal strength at rest, but after fasting or exercise they may show evidence of muscle damage with a raised CK and occasionally myoglobinuria. Carnitine is synthesised only in the liver and is taken up by muscle from plasma. Muscle biopsy may show large fat droplets in the muscle fibres.

11.10 Myotonic syndromes

Myotonia is the slow or delayed relaxation of muscle after a contraction. It differs from the slow relaxation seen in conditions such as hypothyroidism or in fatigued muscle in that the EMG shows that relaxation is accompanied by continuing electrical activity which originates in the muscle fibre membrane (Fig. 11.12).

Myotonia occurs in a number of human muscle disorders of which myotonia congenita is probably the best understood. Myotonic stiffness affects the limb muscles and a common complaint by patients is that they have difficulty in releasing their grip on hand tools. It is a feature of all myotonic conditions that they tend to be aggravated by the cold. The first important step in understanding this condition came through studying myotonia in the goat.

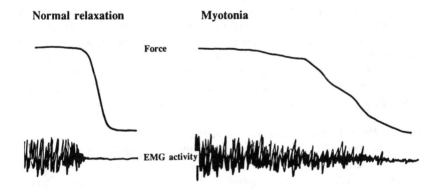

Fig. 11.12 Myotonic discharge and slow relaxation.

The main abnormality in myotonic goat muscle is an increased membrane resistance as a consequence of a reduced chloride conductance. Observations on biopsy specimens of intercostal muscles from human patients with myotonia congenita have shown similar changes. In muscle fibres with a reduced chloride conductance each action potential is followed by a significant after-potential which is cumulative during a train of impulses and is sufficient to induce repetitive firing in the absence of a large chloride leak conductance.

The myotonia of myotonic dystrophy is of a different origin and is probably associated with changes in the resting potential of the muscle membrane.

11.11 The periodic paralyses

The familial periodic paralyses (FPP) are rare disorders characterised by periodic attacks of weakness. There are two main types which give rise to similar muscular symptoms but have quite different causes.

11.11.1 *Hypokalaemic periodic paralysis*

Hypokalaemic periodic paralysis is an autosomal recessive condition which is sometimes associated with thyrotoxicosis. Presentation is most common during the second decade of life when attacks of weakness, which may progress to flaccid paralysis, occur, often during the night. Attacks are precipitated by carbohydrate meals, especially if these are taken after exercise. Giving insulin will also provoke an episode of paralysis. These attacks, regardless of the cause, can be aborted by 10 to 15g of oral potassium chloride or potassium citrate.

Characteristically the weakness is accompanied by a fall in plasma potassium (values as low as 1.5 mM have been reported). This potassium is not lost to the body but moves into the skeletal muscles. It is now generally accepted that the paralysis is accompanied by a large depolarisation of the muscle membranes; evidence comes from recordings *in vivo* and *in vitro*. Relief of paralysis by oral KCl is accompanied by repolarisation of the muscle fibres. The disorder is associated with some abnormality in the transport of K^+ and glucose into the muscle.

11.11.2 *Hyperkalaemic periodic paralysis*

It was found that treating some patients with periodic paralysis with potassium salts made the condition worse. Investigation of this phenomenon lead to the description of hyperkalaemic periodic paralysis. This condition generally presents in the first decade; attacks are provoked by potassium and can be relieved by glucose and insulin. In these respects the condition is the reverse of hypokalaemic periodic paralysis. During attacks, plasma potassium may rise with potassium moving out of the muscles and possibly also from other tissues.

Acetazolamide has proved effective in the long-term treatment of both types of periodic paralyses. It appears to act by reducing potassium fluxes across the muscle membranes.

11.12 Malignant hyperpyrexia

Malignant hyperpyrexia is a rare condition but one that presents considerable problems for anaesthetists. It was first described in Australia in the 1960s. Apparently healthy individuals undergoing routine surgery can develop an alarming and often fatal hyperpyrexia. Typically, after anaesthesia is induced, muscle stiffness is noted in the patient accompanied by a rapid rise in body temperature, an increase in plasma potassium and lactate, and subsequent cardiac failure. Unless the signs are recognised early during anaesthesia and treatment begun promptly, prognosis is poor, death resulting in about 50% of cases. Myoglobinuria and renal damage are additional problems for patients who survive the acute episode. It is now clearly established that the precipitating factors are the use of *halothane* as an anaesthetic agent and/or *suxamethonium* as a muscle relaxant. These substances can potentiate the release of calcium in normal skeletal muscle, as does caffeine. In susceptible individuals this effect seems to be dangerously exaggerated. Treatment is with *dantrolene*, a substance that reduces calcium release from the sarcoplasmic reticulum.

Inheritance is autosomal dominant although the reported incidence is twice as high in males as in females. The incidence has been variously reported as from 1 per 20,000 to 1 per 200,000 persons subjected to anaesthesia. This apparent difference in incidence probably represents differing anaesthetic procedures in the UK and other countries.

The management of susceptible patients requires careful monitoring of body temperature and the avoidance of known precipitating agents and stress. If a hyperpyretic attack develops, intravenous dantrolene should be administered and strenuous efforts made to limit the rise in body temperature.

A condition similar to human hyperpyrexia has been described in Pietran and Landrace pigs. These animals develop muscle rigidity, acidosis and hyperkalaemia, and die of heart failure in stressful conditions. The disease is of considerable economic importance in Denmark and other pork-producing countries because meat from such animals tends to go into rapid contracture post mortem, extruding water and leaving a pale and unattractive product. As in humans, susceptible pigs are sensitive to halothane and depolarising muscle relaxants.

11.13 Summary

Figure 11.13 presents a summary of muscle disorders in which the classification has been based on the the features which are of interest to a clinical physiologist, namely weakness, fatigue or altered function. Inevitably there are conditions where there is an overlap of symptoms, for example, myasthenia gravis and some of the glycogen storage diseases, where weakness and fatigue may both be present. There is, perhaps, little intrinsic value in attempting to classify muscle disorders but we hope that this summary may, at least, become an aid to memory.

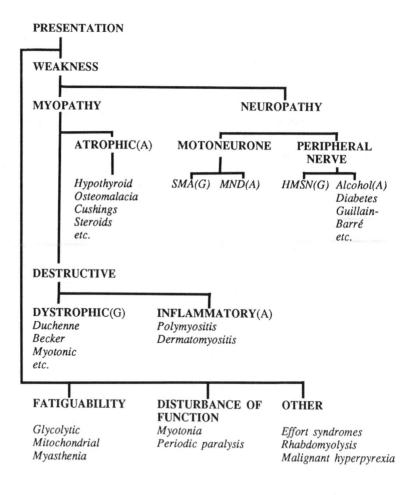

Fig. 11.13 Summary of muscle disorders. (G) indicates a genetic disorder, (A) an acquired disorder; SMA, spinal muscular atrophy; MND, motor neurone disease; HMSN, hereditary motor and sensory neuropathy.

11.14 **References and further reading**

Anderson, J. (1985). *Atlas of Skeletal Muscle Pathology.* Lancaster, MPT Press.

Bohan, A. & Peters, J.B. (1975). Polymyositis and dermatomyositis. *New England Journal of Medicine* **292**, 344-47.

Dubowitz, V. (1985) *Muscle Biopsy: a Practical Approach.* 2nd edition. London, Ballière Tindall.

Edwards, R.H.T. & Jones, D.A. (1983). Diseases of skeletal muscle. In: *Handbook of Physiology, Section 10, Skeletal muscle.* ed. L.D. Peachey, R.H. Adrian & S.R. Geiger, Bethesda, American Physiological Society, pp. 633-72.

Engel, A.G. (1987). Molecular biology of end-plate diseases. In: *The Vertebrate Neuromuscular Junction; Neurology and Neurobiology*, Vol. **23** ed. M.M. Salpeter. New York, Alan R. Liss, Inc., pp. 361-424.

Harding, A.E. (1989). The mitochondrial genome - breaking the magic circle. *The New England Journal of Medicine* **320**, 1341-43.

Hoffman, E.P., Monaco, A.P., Feener, C.C. & Kunkel, L.M. (1987). Conservation of the DMD gene in mice and humans. *Science* **238**, 348-50.

Kunkel, L.M. *et al* (1986). Analysis of deletions in DNA from patients with Becker and Duchenne muscular dystrophy. *Nature* **322**, 73-5.

Morrow, J. & Isenberg, D. (1987). Polymyositis. In: *Autoimmune Rheumatic Disease.* Oxford, Blackwell Scientific Publications, pp. 234-55.

Walsh, F.S., Pizzey, J.A. & Dickson, G. (1989). Tissue-specific isoforms of dystrophin. *Trends in Neurosciences* **12**, 235-38.

Walton, J.N. (ed.) (1981). *Disorders of Voluntary Muscle.* 4th edition. London, Churchill Livingstone.

INDEX